The Family Jewels

A Guide to Male Genital

Play and Torment

by Hardy Haberman

greenery press

Cover photo: Craig Maxwell Photography

Illustrations: Issac Tucker

Published in the United States by Greenery Press, 1447 Park Ave., Emeryville, CA 94608, www.greenerypress.com.

ISBN 1-890159-34-4

Table

of

Contents

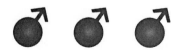

Acknowledgments

No book like this is ever a solitary effort. I have included information and techniques I learned from not only personal experience, but from the wisdom and experience of others, both tops and bottoms. I am very grateful to Janet Hardy at Greenery Press for recognizing the need for a book like this, to Bert Hermann for his gracious referrral, and to my editor Hanne Blank for helping me organize my ramblings.

I would also like to acknowledge the special support of my boy and partner Patrick, who has been a patient friend during the writing and sometimes a test pilot for new techniques and toys. Additionally, a special thank you goes to my many mentors in the Dallas leather community and to that wonderful bunch of wild men of the Chicago Hellfire Club for putting on their annual SM rodeo known as Inferno.

Last but certainly not least a special belated thank you to the late Tony DeBlase, a real master of CBT who was always willing to generously share his experience and time.

Foreword

by

Fetish Diva

Midori

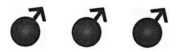

To novice players and curious readers...

It seems counterintuitive. Why would a man want scary and intense things done to such a delicate part of his body? How could this possibly be pleasurable? How could he ask a lover or a playmate to do these seemingly unloving acts to him? If he's asked you, how on earth can you do it to a person you care for? Or, how can you ever ask that special person to do such things to you?

These are some of the questions that may come to your mind when you hear words and images like "cock and ball torment," "genital bondage," "ball stretchers," "pinwheels," "electro-torture"... a pretty intimidating list!

Let me be the first to assure you that it's quite normal to feel a bit intimidated. Let me also assure you that there's nothing wrong with a person finding erotic pleasure in these activities.

The key lies in the subjective nature of sexual pleasure. We all experience and process pleasure and pain uniquely: one man's pleasure is another man's agony. One person might love a very spicy gumbo, while another would find it unbearable and indigestion-inducing. One fellow finds great joy and a physical high from running a marathon, while another would find that beyond the pale. It's the same when it comes to the pursuit of sensual satisfaction. The human experience of pleasure just can't be placed on an absolute scale that's meaningful from one person to another. So, for a moment, let's just let go of all these scary words and intimidating images...

Instead, what if I told you that this book possesses the key to unsurpassed pleasure for some men? What if I told you that you'll learn what makes these men erotically tick in these pages? What if this book could amp up your sensual dominance and deepen his surrender to you? Then might you consider setting aside some initial discomfort to share in the knowledge of an experienced player?

If so, I welcome you to read this book. You'll find a wealth of information shared in an easy conversational style from a vastly experienced player. I want you to consider Hardy Haberman as your amiable guide to new inspirations and sensations. While his tone is approachable and light, he's very thorough and responsible in covering the essential information. You'll learn about the anatomical terrain with a focus on pleasure, sexual response and SM play.

Being a female dominant, and thus lacking in-the-body knowledge of the cock-&-balls response, I find the information shared by male players, whether top or bottom, essential to my development as a skilled player. I believe in experiencing what the bottom will feel before I venture into playing with new activities... but some things are just not feasible!

In the arena of technical information, you'll learn about a full range of play from the easy and relatively mild to the technically demanding and intense. Please note that you are not necessarily expected to progress from the mild to the wild. You may find that you like some of the milder things and will never go to the heavier activities. You may find one intense scene arousing and find the softer scenes not spicy enough for you. This is completely natural: while I very much enjoy CBT, it's likely that I will not do or enjoy all the things that Mr. Haberman covers in this book. Even so, it's interesting to read about them, especially since Mr. Haberman sheds light on the internal experience of the players as well as the recipe for the physical activity.

The material covered in this book is not the entirety of CBT. The human mind is endlessly creative, especially when it comes to matters of pleasure and gratification. Take the knowledge shared here and create your own repertoire of CBT play. With the foundation gained from this book, you'll have a new appreciation for other types of CBT play that you might encounter, or allow you to see potential for play in the common objects. Most of all, you'll appreciate the emotional effect that the range of play can create.

To experienced players….

Whether tops or bottoms, we're always on the lookout for new ideas, aren't we? You'll enjoy this book as you would a cozy post-party chat with another CBT enthusiast. As an erotic sadist who enjoys genital play with both men and women, I found some fresh ideas as well as interesting twists on old familiar equipment in this book. I even found ideas that translated well to female genital play. I'm happy to report that the result of experimentation and implementation of these new ideas on my submissives were quite successful!

Mr. Haberman celebrates the joy of CBT for both the top and the bottom. What the bottom gets out of CBT may be apparent to many SM players. He enjoys erotic pleasure and sensual attention focused around these highly nerve-rich and responsive organs. He is bathed in the full focus of the top. He has a physically and emotionally great time. The pleasure of the top, however, is not always so obvious. For this reason it's a delight to read this book that acknowledges the dominant's thrills – the emotional connection, exercising erotic sadism and taking control of the bottom's ecstasy.

For me, it is a great joy to feel the physical manifestation of my sweet sensual power as I slowly and firmly grasp my lover's balls and squeeze... feeling the direct response to my sexual control over them in their moans and sighs.

Introducing CBT to a partner....

As we noted earlier, sometimes the most difficult thing in SM adventures may not be the technicality or the physical experience of play. It's often the first step of discussing play with potential partners. Many people fear that disclosing a non-traditional sexual interest to a partner may result in misunderstanding, rejection or disgust. Rest assured, it doesn't have to be that way.

Find out first what kind of knowledge and preconceived notions your potential play partner might have on the topic of alternative sexual adventures, SM and even CBT. Be open-minded and be prepared to answer any questions they might have on the topic.

This book can be an excellent point of departure for a discussion on CBT. Remember, however, that you can't just hand a person a book and expect them to fully embrace or appreciate the concepts presented within. Books can be a wonderful reference or starting point in a new adventure, but do not in any way replace the actual experience or physical practice.

If your partner doesn't have the time or inclination to delve into a book, then you can do the reading and personally present and talk about the concepts. Make sure to listen and acknowledge what their reluctance or fears might be.

When it comes to actual playtime, don't overwhelm them by expecting the sun and the moon and all the possible wonderful and amazing CBT experiences you've ever dreamed of. Take it slowly and simply. Have them try one new CBT activity combined with known pleasurable activities. Everyone starts off as a novice. Be patient and generous in spirit if they seem awkward or hesitant. Take the time to discuss your experiences after the scene. Make sure to let them know that you appreciated their adventurous spirit and share with them the fun you had. Ask them if they had fun, and what they found pleasurable about the experience. Remember to be supportive and open-minded. Your patience and understanding will surely be rewarded with shared adventures and wonderful new pleasures.

Wishing every reader of this book many happy and pleasurable moments...

Fetish Diva Midori

You Want To Do *What* To Your Genitals?!?: a gentle introduction to cock and ball play

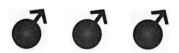

The notion of cock and ball play, or producing a range of non-traditional sensations and feelings in the male sexual anatomy for the purpose of sexual stimulation, often leaves people completely stunned. Why would anyone want to do such things to his genitals? When I first came out into the leather scene, I was under the impression that cock and ball play was practiced solely among gay leathermen like myself. Now I konw better. I suppose my misunderstanding happened because whenever I mentioned any nontraditional or BDSM play involving the "family jewels" to my straight male friends, they would cringe and cross their legs.

It's not an uncommon reaction. Many people just can't make sense of why or how all these various types of sensation and activity (some of which are, yes, painful) could be fun.

For those of us who are drawn to cock and ball play, on the other hand, the urge to experience a wide variety of sensations, some of them extreme, seems like second nature. Many men, myself included, begin to experiment with alternative – by alternative, I mean alternatives to the fairly everyday, typically orgasm-oriented realm of fucking, sucking, handjobs, and masturbation – ways of stimulating their genitals at fairly early ages. One of my favorite masturbation tricks as a teenager was to use the cardboard core from a roll of toilet paper as a sheath around my cock, doing my best to stimulate myself through its tan cardboard walls, titillated by the way it made my own touch seem foreign, as if someone else were touching me. From my vantage point as an adult who has taught cock and ball play workshops for the past six years, I can see that I was using my toilet paper roll as a a basic chastity device, something to prevent me from feeling anything more than the faint pressure of my hand... and I can still remember what an outrageous turn-on it was, too.

For those of us who are attracted to cock and ball play, in other words, finding alternative ways to produce exciting sensations in our genitals is something that in many cases is a pretty intrinsic part of who we are sexually. Men who like cock and ball play may be gay, bi-sexual, straight, pansexual, or celibate (not having sex with partners). Some cock and ball play fans are active members of the BDSM community, some are not, and some may not consider what they do to be BDSM at all. Some like playing with a partner, others really prefer their cock and ball explorations to be a solo thing.

Some people who are interested in cock and ball play don't have cocks and balls. Women, as well as transgendered and intergendered people of any number of types of genital anatomy, may be interested in cock and ball play either for their partners' sakes, or because they are interested in modifying the techniques for use on different types of genitals. As a workshop leader, I find that interest runs high in every community with which I come into contact. I have even had lesbian tops attend my workshops in an effort to better understand how some of the techniques I use can be applied to their female partners. Each time I talk to a new group of people, I meet people I never would've expected, all brought together by our mutual interest in exploring the fun we can have with our naughty little nerve endings.

That's part of the rationale behind this book. Cock and ball play may be outside the mainstream, but given the number and variety of people interested in it, it's certainly not as far outside as all that. Still, it can be hard to find reliable information. I remember that when I was coming out into the BDSM world, the only material I could find on the subject in print was in gay male publications like Larry Thompson's *Leatherman's Handbook* and Tony DeBlase's *Dungeonmaster Magazine*. Until now there has been no single book on the subject to inform the curious, educate the neophyte, and inspire the experienced. Given the popularity of cock and ball play, and given the fact that it is something that can cause damage if not done sanely and with an awareness of potential risks, it seems only sensible that there be some reference on the topic. Besides, having good information and an inspiring example or three at hand might just inspire a few people to take the plunge and move their cock and ball fantasies into reality. More pleasure in the world is hardly a bad thing.

So, just what is it that people do to a man's genitals that constitutes cock and ball play? Lots of things! Cock and ball play can range from something as mild as a tight squeeze of the penis to intense scenes with specialized equipment. It could be a guy who likes to have his partner gently squeeze and twist his balls during oral sex, or a guy who adores nothing more than having a naughty "nurse" or "doctor" clamp a selection of skillfully placed hemostats (perhaps fresh from the ice bucket!)

on his scrotum, a guy who wears a cock ring under his jeans because he likes the heaviness of the metal circle around the base of his equipment, or a gent who loves to ride the endorphin waves of prolonged bondage with weights suspended from his balls under the guidance of a skilled mentor-top. The variety available in cock and ball play is as wide as the spectrum of people who have cocks and balls to play with.

Cock and ball play, in short, involves bringing the desired sensations to the bottom through the direct application of stimulus to the genitals, sometimes in conjunction with genital bondage. All the "traditional" BDSM play types – flogging, sensation play, compression, constriction, electrical play, and many more – are things that can be done in cock and ball play as well. Many all-purpose BDSM toys, and even household implements, can be wonderful tools for cock and ball scenes. There are also a number of toys made and sold specifically for this type of play, many of which are discussed in "The Toy Box" later on, and the toy fancier will find a rich array of choices for his or her collection, capable of delivering sensations from the subtle to the shockingly severe.

That said, cock and ball play certainly doesn't have to be painful. But the boundaries between pain and pleasure often become very blurred during this kind of play, as they do in much sex play. Remember the song "Hurts So Good"? That's precisely the paradox that makes cock and ball play so enjoyable for so many people. Some of the people who are attracted to this kind of play are undeniably masochists, people for whom pain is pleasurable, but that's certainly not always the case. Some people in the BDSM community use cock and ball play as a rite of passage, a symbolic event that marks their transition from a light to a heavy player. Some people use genital play as a route to what I like to call a "peak experience," a metaphysical high that can be reached through the mental and physical concentration and endorphins that are part and parcel of an intense bodily experience. Long-distance runners often talk about the "runner's high." Women giving birth as well as people sitting through long tattoo or piercing sessions often talk about feeling very similar senses of elation and transcendence. Many indigenous peoples have age-old rituals designed to produce these feelings as part of religious or cultural ceremonies. Cock and ball play is just one more possible route to the same place.

A good cock and ball play session can be many things. It can be a finale to a long, involved BDSM scene, or a terrific prelude to a night of hot sex. It can be part of a punishment scene for a naughty boy, or a big reward for an attentive sub. Whether it's mild or intense, cock and ball play is a great addition to any BDSM player's bag of tricks. It may not be the perfect thing for every occasion, but under the right circumstances, it's dynamic, riveting, and passionate. It's exactly this intensity that makes cock and ball play something that can deepen BDSM play experience with a partner or make it more intimate. What might start as a casual play relationship can become deeper when the genitals are directly involved.

Cock and ball play might also be a way for a longterm couple to add an exciting new realm of sexuality to their relationship. I once did a teaching scene with a straight couple for whom cock and ball play was just that. The domme, a relative newcomer to the BDSM world, wanted to learn about cock and ball play as a way of enhancing her sex life with her submissive husband, who had expressed interest in being topped that way. Wisely, they didn't want to jump into cock and ball play without any information, so we had a lengthy negotiation session over coffee, discussing safety and limits before we actually started any action. I assured them both that their limits would be respected, and that the entire scene was really under the domme wife's control, with me being there more as a teacher and as an instrument of her wishes than as a top in my own right. That set the scene, psychologically, for her husband to feel safe, relaxed, and open to fully experiencing everything we tried. It was a great experience for both them and myself, and they seem very happy having added cock and ball play to their sex life together – they've even asked me to expand their play and coach them in some new techniques.

Not everyone who decides to experiment with cock and ball play will need to seek out a private tutor, as the couple I described above decided to do. But still, for most of us, this kind of activity isn't the kind of thing you do on a first date. Cock and ball play scenes need to be negotiated, and the expectations of all the people involved should be discussed beforehand. Part of the fun for me is laying the plans, doing the negotiations, setting the stage for a scene both psychologically and physically, even to the point of building the toys and assembling the props. Cock and ball play isn't just about cocks and balls!

In fact, most cock and ball scenes don't start out focused specifically on the genitals, even though that is where things are going to end up. Getting everyone in the right mood might take a considerable amount of warm-up play. Like most BDSM scenes (and most sex in general) things begin slowly, then gradually intensify, letting the person on the receiving end of the stimulation have a chance to get used to the sensations and the arousal. As I mentioned earlier in this introduction, people tend to experience sensations differently when they're sexually aroused (that "hurts so good" phenomenon). That nifty little mindflip can make things which might be intolerable under other circumstances be very desirable, in the right psychological, physiological, and interpersonal contexts. You wouldn't want a stranger to bite you on the neck, for example, but when a lover does it in the heat of sexual passion, it's likely to be delightful. Cock and ball play is much the same way.

Aside from physical sensation, cock and ball play offers incredible physical and psychological intimacy. That intimacy is one of the biggest turn-ons for me as a top. I think most people are in some way deprived of touch, especially non-transactional touch. What I mean by "non-transactional touch" is this: people rarely get to come into contact with another person's genitals without a specific expectation in mind, such as "I touch you there, therefore we are going to have sex."

In a cock and ball play scene, I can play with another man's most intimate body parts without the *quid pro quo* of traditional genital sex. We can have a very sensual scene and neither of us may reach orgasm. It isn't a necessary part of a scene, and many cock and ball play sessions don't include it. Many times the bottom is exhausted after all the physical and emotional ups and downs of a scene, so an orgasm is simply not a top priority. Other times, it becomes the reward for a good scene. Occasionally, orgasm – or, rather, the withholding of orgasm – can become the scene itself. Taking a partner to the brink of ejaculation and stopping, bringing them back down, then starting again, is a rollercoaster approach to sexual energy. When the orgasm finally does arrive after all that, it's often earthshaking.

But the simple fact is that cock and ball play doesn't require orgasm at all to be earthshaking, and even though it may in a given instance be orgasm-focused or used as foreplay to other types of sex, cock and ball play is also an entity unto itself. The play and the touching themselves can provide such unusual and wonderful feelings for both top and bottom that they are an experience quite beyond more traditional sex. It isn't often you can relate to someone so directly through contact with their genitals when the contact isn't explicitly related to genital sex, an intimacy I cherish and on which I thrive.

Embarking on an exploration of cock and ball play can feel a little like tumbling down the rabbit hole into Wonderland. It's full of amazing and wonderful things, but also includes things that sometimes make even those of us who are quite enthusiastic about alternative forms of sexuality sit and scratch our heads with the same "you want to do WHAT to your genitals?" look on our faces that seems to be the default reaction for people who don't understand its appeal at all. Not every single aspect of cock and ball play is going to work for every single person who is interested in cock and ball play in general, and that's perfectly fine. If you come across some type of play that just doesn't toast your personal Pop-Tarts, don't worry about it. We all have our limits. You're no less of a man, bottom, top, or human being for it.

By the same token, if you dream up or become interested in a type of play that isn't covered in these pages, by all means, experiment, but do it cautiously, sensibly, sanely, and consensually. No matter what you're learning, it's always a fine idea to learn from someone with experience, and this is particularly true with regard to certain types of cock and ball play that have the potential to be physically risky, such as play piercing and any urethral play. If you want to do this kind of thing, make some contacts in the BDSM community and find someone to teach you. Doctors learn how to do these things through hands-on instruction, and you probably should too. There are some things you just can't learn from a book!

When all is said and done, cock and ball play can be a truly extraordinary venue for plumbing the depth and breadth of your own sexuality, with or without a partner. Anyone with a cock and balls to play with already has all the equipment he needs to start experimenting with what can be an extraordinary range of sensations and experiences. Even if you decide not to experiment, just reading and learning is a great way to expand your awareness and knowledge of sexual expression and sexual creativity. The next time someone's got that "you want to do *what* to your genitals?!?" look on their face, you can just nod and smile, knowing that just because cock and ball play isn't everyone's cup of tea doesn't mean it can't be a sublime treat indeed.

1.

The Family

Jewels:

Basic Male

Anatomy

♂ ♂ ♂

I'm not a doctor, but as a top who engages in cock and ball play, I do end up playing one in the dungeon. Before anyone gets started in cock and ball play, it's a good idea to get a better grasp on the materials at hand... sorry, I couldn't resist the pun. What I meant to say is that before you start playing with it, it's a good idea to become well informed about the male sexual, reproductive, and urinary anatomy.

The following is a rough roadmap to all the treasures to be found between the legs of your average guy. It is not intended to replace competent treatment, care, or information from a medical professional. If you, or someone you play with, has any medical or anatomical issues that may be of concern, consult a doctor before engaging in cock and ball play. Dr. Charles Moser's book *Health Care Without Shame: A Handbook for the Sexually Diverse and Their*

Caregivers offers wonderful advice on how to approach sexual issues with your doctor.

The Penis

The penis has five major surface landmarks: the shaft, the glans or head, the corona, the frenum, and the urethral meatus. The shaft is just that, the shaft or stem of the penis. The glans, or head, is the helmet-like or mushroom-shaped head of the penis. The corona is the ridge at the bottom of the glans, and may be more or less definite or large depending on the man. The frenum is the area just below the glans on the underside of the penis, where the ridge of the corona forms a slight point toward the tip. Just under that small "point" is the frenum, which in many men is a particularly sensitive part of the penis. In men who are uncircumcised, the region just below the head of the penis is the point at which the prepuce, or foreskin, attaches to the shaft of the penis. The urethral meatus is the opening at the tip of the urethra, roughly in the center of the head of the penis, also known as the pee-hole.

This leads us to the internal architecture. There's much more to the average penis than meets the eye. Connected to the urethral meatus is the urethra (see illustration). The urethra is the tube through which pre-ejaculatory fluid, semen, and urine all exit the body.

To either side of the urethra, likewise running the length of the penis, there are two long tubes of soft sponge-like tissue. The corpus cavernosum runs along the top, and the corpus spongiosum runs along the urethra. These run the length of the penis, and are basically reservoirs for blood. When these spongy structures are filled with blood, which is a normal part of male sexual arousal, the penis becomes erect. This process is called vasocongestion. Penises do not have to be erect to feel sexual pleasure, though, and lack of an erection does not necessarily mean that a man is not enjoying himself.

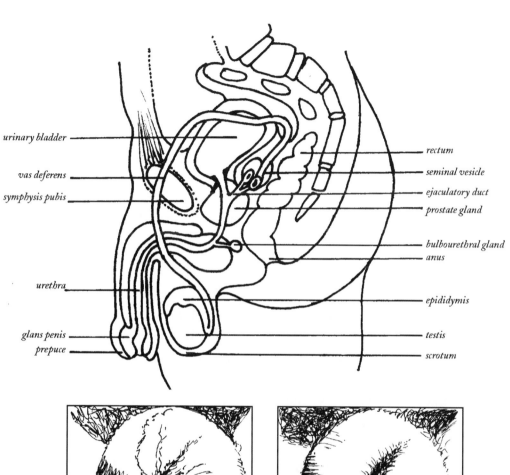

urinary bladder ———————————————— rectum

vas deferens ———————————————— seminal vesicle

symphysis pubis ———————————————— ejaculatory duct

prostate gland

bulbourethral gland

anus

urethra ———————————————— epididymis

glans penis ———————————————— testis

prepuce ———————————————— scrotum

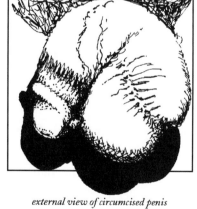

external view of circumcised penis

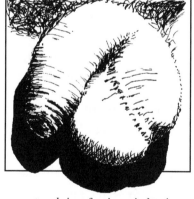

external view of uncircumcised penis

The Testicles

The testicles have two primary exports that are, to many people, the very essence of being male: testosterone (also produced by the adrenal glands) and sperm. They are located inside the scrotum and are semi-hard, basically spherical or oval-shaped bodies that can move around to some degree within the loose skin of the scrotum, a handy feature that helps keep them from becoming injured if squeezed or struck. Squeezing a testicle itself can be potentially harmful, and should be done very gently and with extreme care. The same is true of the epididymis (see below) and vas deferens (see below), ducts which help to transport semen from the testes.

It is normal for one testicle to hang lower than the other. If you notice this in yourself or a play partner, don't be alarmed.

The Scrotum

The scrotum is the "sack" that holds the testicles. It is made of skin and a thin but very flexible layer of muscle. It hangs below the penis, and has a thin dividing layer of muscle tissue, the testicular septum, between its two halves, keeping each testicle in its own compartment. Externally, the two halves of the scrotum are divided by a thin ridge called the raphe. The scrotum is often of a darker skin color than surrounding areas, and its skin contains a high concentration of sweat and oil glands as well as hair follicles. The scrotum often tightens or 'shrinks' when it is cold, during physical exercise, or as part of a fear, nervousness, or arousal reaction.

The Foreskin

The foreskin is a loose tube of penile skin that extends from just below the glans of the penis up and over the head, covering the head of the penis. The foreskin can be rolled back to expose the glans; some men's foreskins retract themselves to some degree when the penis is erect. Circumcision is the process in which the foreskin is removed. Performed on the majority of male babies born in North American hospitals, it means that men with foreskins are in the minority in North America, although they are in the vast majority throughout the rest of the world.

The Bladder

Not technically part of the genitals, but connected so directly as to warrant a mention. The bladder is the place where urine is stored after being filtered out by the kidneys, and it is located slightly above and behind the penis toward the spine. The urethra (see below) is the duct that goes from the bladder to the outside world. Any infections or damage to the urethra can have their repercussions to the bladder, which can cause bladder infections or, if left untreated, kidney infections or other damage.

The Urethra

The urethra carries the urine or semen to the outside of the body. In men, the urethra is about eight inches long. It emerges from the bladder, then passes through the prostate gland (which surrounds the urethra – imagine the urethra as a straw that goes through a "doughnut hole" in the prostate). The seminal vesicles and secretions from the prostate empty into the urethra as well, which is how semen gets into the urethra. The urethral sphincter, a band of muscle, controls the flow of urine into the penis – this is why it's so hard to pee when you have an erection. The longest section of the urethra is the section between the urethral sphincter and the end of the penis, running the entire length of the penis to the urethral meatus or opening. As far as cock and ball play goes, the urethra is primarily useful for play involving sounds or catheters. The inside of the urethra is very delicate and can be damaged easily. Tearing and/or scarring of the urethra can occur when anything is inserted into it, so great care – and a lot of attention to sterile technique and appropriate equipment – should be used if any objects are to be introduced into the urethra.

The Spermatic Cord

The spermatic cord is a bundle of tubes – think of it like a phone cable housing a number of wires – that supports the testicle. There is one on each side. They are sheathed in connective tissue, and contain arteries and veins that supply blood to the testicle, nerves, and the first section of the vas deferens, and run from the testicle itself to the inguinal ring, the opening in the abdominal wall where the vas deferens enters the abdomen. If the spermatic cord becomes twisted (torsion), the testicle can become irreparably damaged.

The Epididymis

The epididymis is an elongated crescent-shaped structure made up of extremely convoluted squiggly tubes. It is attached to the testicle, and serves as a maturation and holding chamber for sperm once they have been produced in the testicles. At ejaculation, sperm move from the epididymis into the vas deferens, and from there to the seminal vesicles and into the urethra. Unejaculated sperm are retained in the epididymis, where they live approximately 4-6 weeks before dying and being reassimilated into the body much in the same way that dead blood cells are. The epididymis is fragile and easily damaged and can be injured by crushing or twisting. Be careful!

The Vas Deferens

The vas deferens are two ducts, one for each testicle, which transport sperm from the epididymis to the seminal vesicles, where the sperm are stored prior to ejaculation. They also contribute some compounds to the makeup of semen, primarily ergothioneine and fructose. The vas deferens are muscular, though lined with mucous membrane. The muscle helps to move the sperm for ejaculation. The spermatic cords (see above), in which a section of the vas deferens are contained, can become twisted (a condition called torsion) due to injury or accident, causing moderate to severe side effects.

The Seminal Vesicles

The seminal vesicles are the final organs through which sperm are channeled as semen is created prior to ejaculation. Sperm and some other fluids are deposited into the seminal vesicles by the vas deferens. In the seminal vesicles, these become mixed with the fluid produced by the vesicles themselves, a thick fluid that contains fructose, proteins, phosphorus, and prostaglandins, among other things, and which constitutes approximately 60% of the total liquid volume of the semen. (FYI: sperm themselves are only approximately 2-5% of the volume of semen. The rest is various fluids produced by the seminal vesicles, the prostate, and other glands and ducts, so yes, they are important!)

The Prostate Gland

The prostate is a chestnut-shaped organ located directly beneath the bladder, surrounding the urethra. It is approximately one and one-half inches in diameter at its broadest point. The two ejaculatory ducts from the seminal vesicles converge with the prostate, uniting with the urethra at the same point. Prostate fluids, sperm, and fluids produced in the vas deferens and seminal vesicles are all mixed at this point. The prostate contributes somewhere around 30% of the total fluid volume of semen. Prostate fluid is clear and slightly acidic, and contains enzymes, citric acid, sodium, zinc, calcium, and potassium, among other things. After about age 50, most men's prostates increase in size somewhat. Many men enjoy having their prostates stimulated, as well as enjoying the sensation of contraction felt in the prostate region during orgasm.

The Cowper's Glands

The Cowper's glands, also known as the bulbourethral glands, are two pea-shaped glands located just beneath the prostate gland at the beginning of the internal portion of the corpus cavernosa (the spongy bodies that extend into the penis and enable erection). They add mucous and the clear lubricating fluid commonly called pre-ejaculate or "precum," which help to neutralize the pH level of the urethra in favor of the health and welfare of the sperm.

2.

Playing It Safe:

"Torture,"

Pleasure, and

Cock and Ball

Play

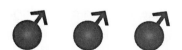

"My God, wouldn't that hurt?" someone who was not in the scene once asked me as I described a particularly nasty piece of cock and ball play equipment.

"Of course," I replied, "it's supposed to!"

The terminology of cock and ball play often includes the word "torture," and is even sometimes referred to as CBT, or cock-and-ball torture. For a lot of people who don't find cock and ball play appealing, the notion of having pain inflicted on the genitals seems like it could be nothing but real, literal torture. To most men, their family jewels are prized possessions. Therefore, cock and ball play – or even the idea of it – can be intensely emotionally threatening to some. That fear can be present even in a willing participant, where it can help put a keen edge on the scene. For others it might inhibit their enjoyment and spoil any mood you might have tried to create, and for still other people, the whole concept is intolerable.

Let's make one thing clear: cock and ball play is not about real torture, even if we might sometimes use the word "torture" as a way to describe it. Real torture is nonconsensual, often creates permanent psychological and physical damage, and is done to hurt people in all senses of the word. Cock and ball play, on the other hand, is consensual, is done to create positive sensations and experiences rather than negative ones, and care is taken not to harm the participants.

And yet, calling it "torture" can still be apt. Cock and ball play, like any form of intense sexual stimulation, can feel torturous – but in the delightful "oh my God I can't take it... it's too much... don't you dare stop" way. As with any BDSM scene, part of the sexual rush comes from the power balance (or imbalance) between the doer and the done-to, the top and the bottom, from the fact that one person is creating sensation and the other person is experiencing it, sometimes struggling to process sensations that are incredibly intense and overwhelming. This, too, can sometimes feel torturous, but in a consensual, mutually pleasurable scene, this "torture" is ultimately overwhelmingly rewarding. It is delightful torture and intense sexual play at the same time.

The point of cock and ball play for me is not to simply inflict pain, but to take my play partner to a peak experience. The sensations I can create in someone's body are a physical means to a metaphysical experience. That metaphysical experience might manifest itself as simply exhilaration and intense arousal, but it might also become an intense release triggering an out-of-body experience. Either way it can be very pleasurable for both parties.

At the same time, it can make a big difference whether cock and ball play is being perceived as "play" or "torture." Depending on which perception applies, a person may be thinking very different thoughts and be inclined toward very different reactions. A top's overt expression of his or her perception of the nature of the play – playful or torturous – is important to put the bottom in the right head space. To an unruly slave or a rebellious boy, a session of cock and ball torture can become a (desired) punishment. To a submissive bottom, genitorture might be endured for the pleasure of the dominant, a show of loyalty and submission. To one boy I play with, cock and ball play is a reward. He loves nothing better than to be strung up and have fifteen to twenty pounds of weight hanging from his balls: to him, cock and ball play is torture only in the most delicious way possible.

Still, cock and ball play can scare the bejesus out of a lot of people. A conscientious player will keep this in mind: it's a good idea to be mindful of how your own play might affect others, particularly if you play in public spaces. I became aware of just how strong some people's fear of cock and ball play can be when I was at a local play party, happily involved in a very heavy cock and ball play session. I had a friend strung up nicely on a rack and was proceeding to hang the last plate of a 25-pound dumbbell set from his scrotum when I heard a timid moan from the corner of the room. Looking over my shoulder, I saw a leather-bedecked Mistress with her two slaves-du-jour cowering naked on the floor, clinging tightly to their Mistress' legs, moaning in absolute and unfeigned terror as they watched my friend and me in our scene. Meanwhile, my play partner was issuing his own moans, but his were the deep, soul-releasing moans of absolute ecstasy. To my friend, it was unimaginably blissful. To the two submissives in the corner, just the sight of it was unimaginably awful. What can I say? There's no accounting for taste!

Safe, Sane, and Consensual

No book on sexuality would be complete without a brief overview of the concept of "safe, sane, and consensual." For many readers, this is probably a very old idea, but the concepts are so essential, and so central to BDSM practice (and indeed, they should be to all sexual activity!) that they bear repeating.

Safe - All parties involved in an act or scene have taken the necessary precautions to ensure that what they are doing will be physically and mentally safe for all concerned.

Sane - All parties involved in an act or scene are in full possession of their mental faculties and understand the risks involved in what they are planning to do. Alcohol and drug use can compromise one's ability to think well and clearly, as well as compromising one's ability to react quickly and well in an emergency: someone who is under the influence of drugs and/or alcohol is not fully "sane" in these senses.

Consensual - All parties understand the potential risks involved in what they plan to do, and agree to what is going to happen and to assuming those potential risks. This consent can be modified or revoked by any person at any time.

Negotiation and Safewords

An important part of keeping things safe, sane, and consensual is negotiation. In brief, this means talking about what you want to do in a scene, or have done to you, what your prior experiences are with the kinds of activity you want to do, and basically getting a good, explicit feeling for what is and is not okay. For the novice, there are many good books about BDSM that go into negotiation in more detail. I recommend Jay Wiseman's *SM 101: A Realistic Introduction* for those who would like more help and advice on how to negotiate a scene, what questions to ask, and how to go about the business of creating useful consensual boundaries for a scene.

For the purposes of cock and ball play, some of the issues you will want to negotiate include:

Types of stimulation: friction, constriction, stretching, impact (slapping, flogging, beating), etc. See page 41 for more categories of play that you may wish to consider when negotiating a scene.

Intensity of stimulation: different people have different levels of sensitivity, and different people find different levels of intensity rewarding. It's a good idea to get some ballpark idea of how intense a sensation might be pleasurable for a given partner before you begin to play. Bear in mind that for some people, successful cock play may involve a different level of intensity from what works for them in terms of ball play, and so on.

Context of play: is the cock and ball play to be done as play, punishment, humiliation, torture, reward, as a meaningful ordeal, or in some other context?

Combining types of play: cock and ball play may be the only ingredient in a scene, or it may be one of several. If you are interested in combining it with other kinds of BDSM play, or with other sex play, you'll want to talk about what things are desirable and okay.

Safewords are words that people use to indicate their status – whether they are okay or not, and sometimes, how they feel more generally – during BDSM play. At minimum, a safeword is a word that a bottom can use to signal the top to immediately stop play in the event that the bottom really needs to stop, if an accident occurs, or simply if a top has hit a limit for that bottom. The word should not be a word that would be used commonly or accidentally during a scene, but should be easily memorable. "Red" is a common safeword, for instance.

Another way of using safewords is to use a "red – yellow – green" system, where a bottom has three safewords that function more or less like the three colors in a traffic signal. The "green" safeword means everything is fine, keep going, the "yellow" safeword means you're getting close to a limit or to a threshold of pain, be careful, and the "red" safeword means stop. Safewords should always be honored without question and as quickly as possible. Tops must be prepared to stop a scene cold if the bottom should happen to safeword, and to be able to release bondage and provide emotional and physical support to the bottom as necessary.

Communication during a scene is by no means limited to safewords. I like to keep up a dialogue between my play partner and myself. By keeping both of us in communication, I keep in touch with how he is processing the stimulation he is receiving. When I do this, I try to make the dialogue part of the scene itself, keeping things more or less in character for the scene: questions are brief and concise, answers are polite and clear. As we have these conversations, I often find that my play partners are willing and sometimes even eager to try something more than they had originally agreed to try. Sometimes, too, I find that they may not be getting quite the desired effect from a scene, and when I know this, I can better adjust to their needs.

As a part of how I like to communicate in scenes, I use a concept that I call "voice" or "scene voice." This principle doubles as a form of safeword, which makes it even more useful. I tend to insist that men who are bottoming to me address me as "Sir," but other special names, titles, or honorifics would work just as well. If at any time during a scene a partner needs to give me information or needs to alter the intensity of a scene, they are told to address me by name instead. That way, we have something that functions very much like a safeword, without the bottom having to remember anything more than my name.

Likewise, I will refer to my partner by a formal submissive title, such as "boy," unless I need to give him information about how I am doing in a scene. People often forget this, but tops need safewords too. Intense scenes can end up putting a top in an uncomfortable place, either psychologically or physically, and sometimes tops as well as bottoms need to adjust or end scenes for their own comfort, safety, and sanity.

In general, I have found using "voice" or "scene voice" to be a very effective method. It allows a free flow of communication during a scene, and can offer more flexibility than a safeword alone. As long as a partner answers my questions in formal "scene voice," I know things are going well, and when I am addressed by name, my ears immediately prick up and I am prepared to listen and respond.

Good Pain vs. Bad Pain

In cock and ball play, perhaps more than any other form of BDSM, the difference between "good pain" and "bad pain" is key. By "good pain," I mean a sensation that, while it may be painful, is felt as positive, that feels good, and that does not cause a type or degree of discomfort that registers automatically as something that is causing harm or that needs to stop. Like scratching a sunburn, good pain is painful and pleasurable at the same time. "Bad pain," on the other hand, is any pain that feels like, well, *pain…* in the sense that it doesn't feel good, it doesn't feel positive, and that registers as something that is causing harm and/or needs to stop.

Sometimes the difference between good pain and bad pain is one of "head space" or mental state. You may, for instance, enjoy being spanked in a BDSM scene when you are turned on and know that you are going to be spanked – that'd be good pain! But you probably wouldn't enjoy being spanked if someone just walked up to you in a nonsexual environment and hit you on the ass without warning. That'd be bad pain, and would be emotionally and socially unpleasant as well.

Sometimes, the difference between good pain and bad pain is the type of pain or sensation, or the degree of pain or sensation. Generally speaking, most people have a pretty good idea of how much pain they can tolerate, and what it feels like when something is going wrong or hurting them. Trusting your instincts – and the instincts of the people with whom you play – is always a good idea.

For some people, there are certain types of pain or sensation that simply do not feel good to them: someone who likes having his cock spanked and would consider that "good pain" might really hate the sensation of having his balls tugged on, and would consider that "bad pain." But the same man, even though he liked having his cock spanked, would very likely have some upper limit to how hard or for how long he was able to process that pain as a positive sensation. When we get tired, or if our mood changes precipitously, good pain can become less than good. Always respect that, and always respect your own boundaries (or those of someone you are playing with) in terms of what is "good pain" or "bad pain" for them. This is true in negotiations as well as when someone uses a safeword.

At the same time, remember that the male genitals are very sensitive and very delicate. As a top, you may have to adjust your perception of what levels of stimulation are appropriate and what is too much. Attention to technique is also important: hitting what you intend to hit in the way you intend to hit it, knowing what's safe in terms of grabbing, tugging, or twisting, and knowing how to troubleshoot potential accidents can make all the difference. A bad hit with a flogger across a back or buttocks will rarely end a scene, but a bad hit or accident during cock and ball play can stop a scene cold. The male genitalia are not called the "family jewels" for nothing, and injuries to the penis and testicles can be irreversible. Even if the injury is not permanent, it can be painful in a way that no one would find fun.

Troubleshooting Physical Play

The primary goal of cock and ball play is pleasure, and lots of it. One of the best routes to making sure that things stay pleasurable is to know what kinds of risks different kinds of play entail. When you know what can go wrong, you have a much better idea of how to steer clear of damage and how to manage things if an accident should happen.

This section discusses the primary types of possible problems and mishaps that could come up during or after cock and ball play. This is not an exhaustive list, but it is fairly representative, and will give you a good idea of what to watch out for and what to do in case something does go wrong.

Impact and Compression Play Risks

Impact play is any play in which something makes impact with or on the cock and/or balls – slapping, hitting, flogging, whipping, et cetera. Compression play is any play that binds, constricts, pinches, smushes, or mashes the cock and/or balls, from tightly winding ropes or cords to pinching with the fingers to using a press or vise and beyond. Cock rings, vacuum pumps, and cock harnesses are related. These kinds of play can cause bruises, welts, edema, and sometimes, phlebitis of surface veins in the cock or scrotum.

Bruising. Bruising happens when capillaries in the skin get broken and there is minor bleeding within the skin. Most superficial bruises will go away on their own in a few days to a week or so. Cold compresses can help limit the extent of a bruise by helping the capillaries to constrict, but if you choose to use ice, make sure you wrap it in a washcloth or towel and remove it if the area feels numb: the last thing you need is frostbite!

Hematocele. This is a variant on bruising, basically, a body of clotted blood that develops in the scrotum following an injury. A lump may be felt, along with external bruising. Small hematoceles often reabsorb without treatment, but large ones often require surgical removal. In general, any lump in the scrotum should be assessed by a doctor.

Welts. A welt is a raised, usually red area of the skin. Welts are most common with whipping and flogging: a thin object, hitting fairly hard, is most likely to raise a welt. Sometimes bruising accompanies a welt. To reduce swelling, you may wish to use a cool or cold compress or a cool water bath.

Phlebitis, a.k.a. Thrombosed Surface Veins. Occasionally, a surface vein in the penis or scrotum will sustain some damage and become hard and painful due to clotted blood within the surface vein. Some swelling of the penis may accompany this. It may take weeks or even months for things to get back to normal. During this time, warm compresses or baths and aspirin or ibuprofen can be helpful to reduce the swelling and clotting. If the phlebitis is persistent or gets worse, see a doctor.

Edema. Edema is swelling of a body part because of injury. If any body part suffers from constricted circulation for a prolonged period, tissue damage may occur. This injury is most common when using something that is very tight around the cock or scrotum: a cock ring, cock harness, ball stretcher, cock and ball bondage. It can be hard to tell if edema is happening in a cock and ball play scene because, well, things do get swollen when men are aroused. A good rule of thumb is to remove any cock or ball bindings every half an hour or so and allow a few minutes to re-establish normal circulation. For this reason, it's not a good idea to leave anything that is binding or tight around the cock and/or balls on overnight. If edema is a constant problem and unrelated to play, or if the swelling doesn't subside within a few hours, see a doctor. [Also see "Removing A Stuck Cock Ring," page 31.]

Twisting and Bending Play Risks

Twisting or bending the cock and/or balls can be very potent! In general, twisting tends to apply to the balls, and bending tends to apply to the penis. Bear in mind that a hard cock is much easier to damage than a soft one, and that the spongy bodies that allow erection extend into the abdomen, so bending the cock counts even if you're bending it where it meets the body. The same is true with twisting the balls. Remember, all this stuff is attached, and we want it to stay that way! This kind of play is really ripe with sensation – a little goes a long way.

Skin stretching or tearing. Sometimes, energetic or intense play means that skin gets stretched or slightly torn. This is particularly common with foreskins and scrotums, where there is loose skin. If the injury is minor, letting it heal on its own is usually fine. A cold compress can help reduce swelling, and aspirin or ibuprofen will help with pain and inflammation. More significant injuries should be seen by a doctor immediately, particularly since any activity vigorous enough to cause skin tearing might damage things other than just skin.

Also, be aware that stretched skin is much easier to puncture than non-stretched skin. If you are playing with skin that is stretched, for instance by a ball stretcher or other device, be extra careful, as the skin will be far more delicate than it would be under other circumstances.

Torsion. Torsion, or twisting, happens to the spermatic cords, bundles of nerves, ducts (including the vas deferens) and blood vessels that link the testicles to the body. Torsion can happen as a result of sex play, but it can also happen during exercise or just at random. Symptoms of torsion are severe pain and swelling in the scrotum, usually along with nausea or vomiting. A twisted spermatic cord cuts off the blood supply to the testicle, and if the cord is not untwisted in time, the man may lose his testicle. If you suspect this has happened, seek medical advice immediately. Doctors have seen this before. Remember to be frank with your doctor. This condition is sometimes misdiagnosed as epididymitis, an infection which causes a similar swelling. Antibiotics prescribed for epididymitis will not help torsion.

Torsion can also happen due to accidents with cock and ball bondage. A friend of mine fell prey to this malady from falling asleep in a very tight ball stretcher. During his sleep, one testicle became twisted.

The minor surgery needed to correct this was not very painful, but the added medical expense and the weeks of abstinence while recovering were not worth it.

Rupture of the Corpus Cavernosa. This is what's known as a penis fracture or "broken dick," and happens when the Tunica Albuginea, the tough membrane surrounding the spongy bodies that fill with blood and enable erection, gets ruptured or broken, usually due to a sudden and very hard blow or bending of the hard penis. Most men who suffer this unfortunate condition hear it happen: there is no bone in the penis, but when the Tunica Albuginea is ruptured, there is often a loud cracking noise, very much like the sound people hear when they break a bone. When this happens, there is immediate pain, severe bruising, and, usually, a fairly immediate loss of erection (no kidding!). This is a serious injury and usually requires surgery. See a doctor immediately.

Bruising. Bruising can also take place with bending and twisting play. Treat as described on p. 25.

Sensation Play Risks

Sensation play is any play that involves touching, stroking, tickling, scraping, or otherwise stimulating the skin of the cock and balls with any number of tools (including body parts like fingers, fingernails, teeth, hair, etc.). The primary risks in sensation play are abrasion and puncture. You can control your risk of injury from sensation play by choosing to play with toys that are less likely to cause heavy friction or puncture, and by paying attention to the condition of the skin as you play.

Abrasion. Abrasions are caused by friction. Mild abrasions often look a bit like sunburn. Heavier abrasions might look like a "skinned knee" type of abrasion, with some crust or a scab forming. Generally speaking, abrasions will take care of themselves if you give them time to heal. You might wish to put a thin layer of a triple-antibiotic cream on an abrasion. Be extra-careful to always use a condom for any genital sex if your skin is abraded, since damage to the skin raises your risk of becoming infected with any STD organism that might be present.

Puncture. Accidental or intentional puncture of the skin alone is usually something that will heal up by itself, kept clean and given time to do so. If deeper tissues have been punctured, see a doctor. The biggest risk with punctures is that of infection. Any toy that might puncture the skin should be a single-user toy for this reason as well as for safer sex reasons, and punctures themselves should be watched for any sign of infection. If a puncture becomes hard, hot, is accompanied by a fever, or is oozing greenish or yellowish pus, see a doctor. Likewise, any deep puncture that results in heavy bleeding should be assessed by a doctor as soon as possible. It is generally okay to puncture skin, as in play piercing, if it's done by a knowledgeable person and with medically sterile equipment. It's not a good idea to puncture tissues below the skin surface, such as the spongy bodies of the penis or the testicles.

Be aware that stretched skin is much easier to puncture than nonstretched skin. If you are playing with skin that is stretched, for instance by a ball stretcher or other device, be extra careful, as the skin will be far more delicate than it would be under other circumstances.

Urethra Play Risks

Play that involves the urethra is particularly risky business because the urethra is so delicate and so easy to injure. This is why only things that are intended for urethral insertion should ever be put into the urethra – urethral sounds and urethral catheters. They should be sterile, too, and insertion should be done with plenty of sterile water-based lubricant. There are plenty of horror stories (many of them backed up with documented medical case histories) about people suffering serious injury, needing surgery, and so forth due to having inserted inappropriate objects into their urethras. Judging from the medical literature, pens, pencils, and toothbrushes are popular problem-causers, so leave the office supplies on your desk and your toothbrush in the bathroom! If you want to do urethra play, educate yourself first about the proper equipment and how to follow sterile procedures when you're playing. Learning in person from a very experienced player is probably your best bet. Your partners will thank you, and so will their penises.

Injury to the Urethra. Injuries inside the urethra can happen if something is inserted into the urethra. Sometimes, this can happen even with extremely careful and practiced players (even doctors and nurses in professional settings sometimes unintentionally injure their patients' urethras) using all the right equipment and doing all the right things: bodies don't always behave the way we expect they will. If there is pain while peeing, blood in the urine, or blood coming from the urethral opening, see a doctor. Even if there is no blood, it's possible for trauma to the urethra to cause scar tissue, too, so be sensitive about how things feel after you engage in urethra play. If you're worried, it's usually best to consult a urologist to be on the safe side.

Urethral Infections. Infections in the urethra, or urethritis, can happen because microorganisms were introduced into the penis through urethra play, unprotected genital sex, or sometimes simply on their own. Typical symptoms are burning while peeing, a cloudy, milky, or greeny-yellow discharge from the urethra, and pain during genital sex. See a doctor for diagnosis and treatment.

Electrostimulation Risks

A primary risk from electrostimulation – even when the electrostimulation is practiced carefully and according to the manufacturer's guidelines for use of electrical toys – is burns. Minor burns can be treated as for abrasions, but anything worse than a first or second-degree burn should be assessed by a doctor. Be careful to read all the manufacturers' guidelines for your electrostimulation equipment before playing, and to educate yourself about the risks of electric play. I recommend *Juice: Electricity For Pleasure and Pain*, by Uncle Abdul, for those who want to learn more.

Ointments, Gels, and Creams Risks

Some people enjoy the sensation of using a sports rub, muscle ache balm like Ben-Gay or Tiger Balm, or similar substances on the skin during cock and ball play. Sometimes, these may cause burning more intense than desired, but because they are oil-based, they can be difficult to remove completely. If you need to remove these creams, or if someone is suffering from an "overdose" of an oil-based cream that's been applied to their skin, wash the area with plenty of warm water and liquid dish soap. Because liquid dish soap is designed to cut oils, it will do a good job of cutting through the oil-based creams as well. Some people also recommend using shampoo and/or witch hazel.

Removing A Stuck Cock Ring

Every once in a while, a man wearing a metal cock ring will become "stuck," unable to remove the cock ring due to the degree of swelling in his penis or scrotum. Before you resort to the bolt cutters or a trip to the emergency room to have the cock ring professionally removed, though, try these tactics first:

- Lie down and wait. If you can be calm, and give your erection a chance to subside, you may well be able to remove the cock ring without a problem.

- Cool the penis and scrotum with a cool water bath or an ice pack wrapped in towels. Bringing down the erection and any additional swelling will often allow you to remove the cock ring yourself.

Other Lumps, Bumps, and Ouches

These are not necessarily due to, or even related to, cock and ball play, but they can influence your genital health and might become a factor in your play. If you or a partner are dealing with any of these conditions, it might be best to postpone cock and ball play at least until you've talked to a doctor about it. For advice on how to approach your doctor about sex play issues, Dr. Charles Moser's book *Health Care Without Shame* is a wonderful resource.

Epididymitis. Inflammation or infection of the epididymis, characterized by a swollen, painful lump inside the scrotum. See a doctor for treatment. Any mass in the scrotum should be assessed by a doctor.

Hydrocele. A collection of fluid in the membrane that houses a testicle. These usually are harmless and painless, but sometimes may get in the way. If they do, see a doctor, since they can be drained. Any mass in the scrotum should be assessed by a doctor.

Orchitis (sometimes called Orchiditis). Infection of a testicle, usually along with severe swelling, pain, and a very swollen scrotum. Any mass in the scrotum should be assessed by a doctor.

Peyronie's Disease. A condition where a scar-like formation of tissue bends the penis in such a way that erection may be uncomfortable or even impossible. No one is sure what causes Peyronie's Disease, and many cases go away as spontaneously and quickly as they arrive. Treatments vary, so consult your doctor.

Prostatitis. An inflamed or infected prostate gland can cause pain, groin pain, frequent urination, fever, and other symptoms, including pain-related impotence. As with any infection, see a doctor.

Variocele. A mass of enlarged veins in the scrotum that can feel like a "bag of worms" to the touch. This is usually harmless, but it might be desirable to see a doctor if it feels uncomfortable or impairs fertility. Any mass in the scrotum should be evaluated by a doctor.

Safer Sex

I just can't write about possible injuries to the male anatomy without some discussion of what has come to be called "Safer Sex." Those two words probably conjure up images of condoms and dental dams, but there is more to safe sex than barrier protection. Sex in general and cock and ball play in particular put both tops and bottoms in situations where bodily fluids might come into play.

Since there are a host of sexually transmitted diseases, including HIV, it is a good idea to know the medical condition of your partner. Talking about sexual history and safer sex practices is always a good idea, and it is also a good thing to talk about specific diseases: is your playmate HIV-positive? Does he have genital herpes (even if there are no active lesions)? How about genital warts, a.k.a. HPV? Does he have chronic or active hepatitis? All these are good questions to ask before getting into a scene.

If you are too timid to ask or talk about these kinds of things, *don't play!* Seriously, I mean that. Among intelligent, consenting, sexually aware adults, having a frank discussion about such important health matters should be something that's expected. A medical condition doesn't have to preclude cock and ball play, but knowing what you're dealing with gives you a much better idea of how to make it a rewarding experience for both of you without life- or health-threatening consequences.

Unless your partner is HIV-positive, or has another disease that might be spread via body fluids, latex gloves are not necessarily required unless you foresee semen, blood or urine as part of the scene. Remember, this is about cock and ball play, not fucking or sucking! For genital sex, always use a condom... and I do mean *always*!

When selecting rubber gloves, check to see if your partner has an allergy to latex. This is a growing problem these days, as some people become allergic after prolonged exposure to latex. If you have ever gotten a rash or inflamed skin while wearing latex gloves, you probably have a latex sensitivity, and should consider using vinyl or hypoallergenic synthetic rubber gloves. They cost a little more, but it's worth it. Any medical supply house will have alternatives to latex exam gloves, and so do many drugstores with good "home health care" sections.

If you choose not to wear gloves – and often, there is no reason you need to – just be watchful for fluid contact. If your partner ejaculates or drips pre-cum during a scene, be careful about where it goes. A little fluid on your hands probably won't matter unless you have cuts or open sores of some kind, but our hands get subjected to a lot, and we often have little injuries like hangnails and paper cuts without really noticing it, so keeping your mitts out of the line of fire is always prudent.

I wear leather gloves during CBT scenes. Leather will not protect against transmission of HIV or other diseases. In fact, the porous nature of leather can trap viruses and bacteria. What to do? Cleaning the gloves well and reconditioning them using leather cleaner is one option, but it is not completely risk-free. An alternative would be to use a different pair of gloves for each partner. This can get expensive, but if you are a top, you can have your bottom bring you a pair of gloves as an offering – a special toy you will use for him only. Kind of sweet, isn't it?

Cleaning Your Toys

Cleanliness is next to godliness, just like Mother always said, and it's a pretty good idea for you, too. Clean toys are more pleasant and a lot safer to play with, so taking care of your equipment – including the inanimate stuff – is important. This is particularly important should your partner ejaculate during a play session, or if there is pre-cum. To avoid transmitting infection, remember to clean up your toys afterward!

Some toys – solid steel toys particularly – won't be harmed by a soaking in a solution of 10% household chlorine bleach and 90% cool water. They can also be boiled to sterilize them. Leather, as mentioned previously, cannot be disinfected completely, but should be cleaned and conditioned with leather cleaner. If you know that you're likely to get bodily fluids on a leather item, making it a one-person toy can be a good safety measure, particularly if you play with partners who are HIV-positive or who have active or chronic hepatitis. Rubber, latex, silicone, and other plastics like vinyl and PVC can be washed with antibacterial soap and plenty of hot water, or run through a cycle in your dishwasher. Silicone toys can also be boiled to sterilize them. Ropes can be washed in the washing machine on hot with a dose of bleach (put them in a lingerie bag or a pillowcase with the end tied shut to help keep things from tangling in the wash).

Some toys, like urethral sounds, should be professionally sterilized in an autoclave. Some tattoo parlors or piercing studios will do this for you for a nominal fee. You can also talk to an experienced urethral-sound player or to a doctor, tattooist, or piercer about how best to make sure your implements stay as sterile as possible until you use them. Catheters are sold in sterile, one-use-only, prepackaged units and cannot be reused.

A note to medical professionals: Please take my use of the term "sterilization" in this book to mean "high level disinfection." Studies have shown that boiling or bleach use alone does not kill all micro-organisms. Only a high-pressure autoclave or gas sterilizer can assure total sterility. However, these machines are generally out of reach of the average BDSM player, and so prudence and caution, coupled with attention to high level disinfection, must suffice in most cases.

Blood Sports. If you are indulging in an activity where the skin is going to be broken, precautions must be more significant and consistent. Always wear medical exam gloves, either latex or a non-latex version. These should be clean, one-use only gloves. If you can get them, sterile surgery gloves are best, but latex exam gloves will suffice if they are kept clean and in the original box.

My preference is a latex exam glove. These are snug enough to allow complete sensation and agility, but provide an effective barrier against possible contamination. The problem with latex is the potential for an allergic reaction. If you notice any complications, switch to non-latex gloves, which will be available in any medical supply store or in a drugstore with a large "home health care" section.

Gloves are very good at preventing an infection or disease organism from passing from one person to another through blood or other bodily fluids that might come into contact with the hands. However, they do not eliminate the possibility of contamination from other sources – from the environment you are playing in to the toys you use – to the person you are playing with. This can be minimized through keeping the site of the play area clean, changing gloves frequently, and using germicidal cleansers.

Items used for blood play need to be as clean as possible, preferably sterile. Hypodermic needles come in one-time-use sterile packaging for precisely this reason. Used needles and other single-use blood play items should be disposed of in hard plastic "sharps containers" to prevent accidental cuts and needle sticks. An empty hard plastic juice jug with a screw-on lid makes an excellent sharps container. You can tape the lid on with packing tape and mark the container "biohazardous waste" for extra security.

Items that are not sterilizable, such as "vampire gloves" – leather driving gloves with sharp, thin metal spikes protruding from the palm and/or fingers – should be single-user toys, to be used on one person and one person only, to avoid the risk of transmitting blood-borne disease organisms.

Psychological Safety

In our culture, men's identity and perception of themselves as men are often at least partially conflated with the presence (and sometimes size) of their cocks and balls. We say that someone "has balls of steel" if they're particularly nervy or courageous, but that they're "dickless" if they're ineffectual or cowardly. Think of how we use words like "emasculated," "castrated," "castrating," and even "effeminate," and you get a pretty good picture of what having a cock and balls often means, not just to a man's sex life, but to the way he's perceived by himself and others.

Hand in hand with this comes our culture's deep fear of castration, a fear that is often more metaphorical than it is actual, but nonetheless one which immediately gets the attention. Add to that the simple fact that almost every penis-owner knows that an accidental or not-so-accidental blow to the crotch means nearly incapacitating pain, and it isn't so hard to understand why the notion of cock and ball play can sometimes put a primal, almost unnamable sense of fear into our heads – and sometimes, that includes the heads of people who practice it. In small doses and tempered by a knowledge that cock and ball play is not about castration or real injury, this fear is a piquant spice that adds some psychological depth to what might otherwise be just another type of sensation play. In larger doses, or if the fear gets too large and uncontrollable, it can cause real terror and outright panic. Good, thorough, honest scene negotiation and frequent checking in with a partner during a scene can help you steer clear of psychological danger points, but sometimes things just happen.

It isn't often that you or a partner will run into a situation where psychological danger becomes a serious issue, or that panic attacks occur, but it's also not completely out of the question for cock and ball play (or indeed for any sexual interaction). The mind is a complicated place, and sometimes things surface during sexual, sensual, or BDSM activity that have been hidden for a lifetime. Should you encounter a situation where someone (you or a partner) begins to have overwhelming feelings or panics during a scene, it's wise to know what to do.

What to do, in almost every case, is to call a time out. Use a safeword if you need to, or simply call a time out to get grounded and do some gentle talking. Remove any bondage and/or toys that may be in use as quickly as you can while being gentle and caring, and reassure the person who is having trouble that everything is okay, that they are in a safe place, and that you are not going to leave them while they are not feeling okay. Have the person sit or lie down, and sit with them as they calm down. Talking is often helpful. Try not to be judgmental, and definitely don't take it personally – in all likelihood, whatever has come up is not about you, but about the situation, and to some degree about that person's own personal quirks and history. The most important things to do are to take it easy, provide a comfortable, safe space, and to get the person grounded enough that he feels more or less back to normal.

In all my years of being a cock and ball player, I have had a serious psychological emergency happen only once. Most of the people I play with are experienced players with a good knowledge of their own internal selves and fears, but having a play partner begin hyperventilating and going into a full-fledged panic attack when we were in the middle of a scene taught me that no matter how self-assured and in control someone may be, these things can still occur. As soon as I noticed that my partner was beginning to hyperventilate, I began to slow down the scene to give him more time to adjust to it. I gave that a few moments, but when that didn't seem to work, I simply whispered in his ear that he was being a very good "boy" and that I was going to reward him. At that point, I gently removed his bondage, reinforcing to him that he was being good and that everything was okay and suggesting that he try to breathe slower and relax. I caressed his face, removing the focus from his genitals. Soon, my play partner began breathing more normally, and, encouraged by my calmness and my own slow breathing, he soon began to feel a lot better. Once my partner had calmed down physically, a process which took about fifteen minutes, we began talking about what he had been feeling. As we talked, I held him close and focused on nurturing and caring for him, and the session ended with both of us feeling good, despite the fact that a psychological emergency had ended the play.

Nurturing is an excellent skill for a top to have, both for handling emergencies and simply for enhancing your experiences with your partners. The aftercare that follows a scene is as important as the scene itself. The aftercare period is a time that lets both you and your partner(s) come down from the emotional high of a scene, and allows you time for bonding and sharing before you have to begin interacting with the rest of the world.

3.

The Toy Box:

Clamps and

Wax and

Weights and

Creams and

Rings and

Whips...

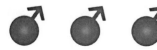

Just as you can't make a good omelet before you know the basic principles and materials of cooking, you can't really create a good cock and ball play scene for yourself or a partner without knowing about basic principles and equipment.

Most cock and ball play, with the exception of the most esoteric practices, falls into one of the following general categories.

Constriction – Any play that constricts the tissues or blood flow. Toys used for this include cock rings, ball separators, ball harnesses, rope, straps, or any genital bondage.

Compression – Play that compresses the cock or balls, sometimes also called "crushing." Some toys used for this are elastic bandages, ball crushers, bar clamps, etc.

Distention – Stretching or spreading the skin, usually of the balls or foreskin (erect penises don't have much spare skin to work with). The toy selection for this type of play includes ball stretchers, stocks, twitches, parachutes, weights, etc.

Percussion or Impact – Any hitting or striking, whether using an implement or the hands/fingers.

Pressure – Clamping, pinching, or otherwise compressing small areas of tissue or skin. Some tools used for this include clothespins, clamps, clips, mousetraps, and forceps.

Puncture – Puncturing the skin superficially as a form of sensation play. One of the kinds of play known as "blood sports." Toys used for this include tracing wheels, Wartenburg wheels, vampire gloves, hypodermic needles and acupuncture needles.

Temperature – Play that involves using heat or cold for sensation. This can also include the use of compounds which do not actually change the temperature, but which give a hot, cold, or "icy hot" sensation when applied to the skin. Some toys used for this are hot candle wax, ice, sports rubs, light bulbs, heating pads, and warm or cold water.

Friction – Friction is a form of sensation play produced by rubbing the cock or balls with any material likely to provide friction, from mild to heavy. Some things that can be used for this are loofahs, fingers, Velcro, brushes, emery boards, burlap, terrycloth, and the rough side of dressed leather.

Teasing & Tickling – Exactly what it sounds like. Fingers, feathers, fur, silk, satin, hair, flower petals... just about anything that would provide a safe, teasing sensation on the skin.

Electrostimulation – Using electricity safely to provide stimulation. It is important to use only devices that are made for this use, as electricity can be dangerous! Toys for this include the Violet Wand, "TENS" units or shock boxes, and other electrostimulation toys designed for sexual use.

Toys, Toys, and More Toys

There are so many options when it comes to toys for cock and ball play that the mind reels! To be honest, you can do cock and ball play without any special equipment at all – it doesn't take anything more than what God gave you – but, as many of us have already learned, part of the fun of BDSM is acquiring and trying out toys.

These days, there is a small industry based on the production sale of cock and ball toys. Leather shops, catalog sales and specialty retailers have long realized the public's fascination with genital devices, and many men and women who have never considered themselves anything but "vanilla" and un-kinky regularly use cock and ball toys. Of these, the cock ring is probably the most familiar. Once sold as a quasi-medical device to help prolong erections by keeping the blood in the penis longer, a cock ring can make an erection feel more intense. There are plenty of variations on the cock ring theme, as well as many unrelated devices, any of which can be used for the pleasure of anyone with a cock, balls, and the will to experiment. Toys are listed here in alphabetical order.

Alligator Clips. These little devils can be found at any hardware or electronics store. They come in a variety of spring strengths and – let this be a warning! – many are too strong to be suitable for cock and ball play. The sharp teeth on some of these clamps can also be a problem, so I suggest trial and error in finding the right kind. This does not involve exposing oneself in the hardware store! The skin webbing between the fingers has about the same consistency as the scrotal sac, though your hands are slightly more resilient than your genitals. Therefore, if you cannot stand the clips on the space between your fingers, you certainly don't want to use them on your nuts!

Ball Separators. Basically a cock ring, but with the addition of a strap which comes from the base of the scrotum (the part of the ring behind the balls) and wraps up and between between the testicles, attaching to the ring at the upper side of the penis. These gadgets look somewhat like tiny athletic supporters. They push the testicles apart and away from the body on the horizontal, rather than vertically in the manner of a ball stretcher.

Ball Stocks. These nice, Spanish-Inquisition-looking things are usually made of wood and act both as a bondage device and a ball stretcher. The balls extend through a hole, and are then constricted by tightening down the halves of the stocks with wing nuts or bolts. Don't pinch the skin of the scrotum in the stocks when you tighten them down!

Ball Stretchers. These are in effect cock rings for the scrotum, a tight leather or rubber strap that constricts the top of the scrotum, pushing the balls away from the body. Since this skin is very elastic, the extent to which the balls can ultimately be stretched can be dramatic. The elasticity of the skin of the scrotum gives stretched balls a shiny smooth appearance, since the skin will be stretched tightly over the testicles themselves.

The psychological effect of ball stretchers can be startling. The body is not used to having the testes so far from the base of the penis. The physical sensation is often one of disconnectedness from the balls, a sort of pseudo-castration. I have one stretcher that is almost 4" in length. This is pretty extreme, and probably would be impossible for some-

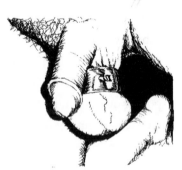

steel ball stretcher

one just starting out. I certainly wouldn't recommend it as a beginner's toy!

Though there is little danger from a scene using a stretcher, leaving ball stretchers on for long periods of time can break down the tissues of the scrotal sac causing permanent distention. Refer to "Impact and Compression Play Risks," page 25, for troubleshooting advice.

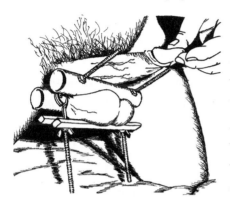

Ball Vise. This nasty-looking specialty gadget has a bar that can be slowly tightened down with wing nuts or bolts in order to compress and "crush" the balls. A recent innovation in the ball vise depeartment is a Plexiglas version, so you can watch the scrotal sac as it flattens out.

ball vise

There should be no need to caution you about this one, but I will anyhow: compression is fine, but actually crushing the testicles causes permanent damage.

Bamboo Skewers. Not for piercing! These thin skewers, usually sold as cocktail skewers, are used in cock and ball play for either teasing or slapping against the balls and penis. Stroking those sharp tips as lightly as you can against the skin gives a sensation a little like walking through a spiderweb. Be careful – these seemingly harmless sticks can really get intense in terms of sensation, and can also raise welts if you hit too hard. Slim knitting needles are another option for similar play and effects. Never insert a bamboo skewer, knitting needle, or other object not intended for urethral use into your (or anyone else's) urethra for any reason.

Blindfold. Blindfolds are great accessories to any BDSM scene. Two things can make cock and ball play even more effective: for a bottom to be able to see absolutely everything that is happening to him, and for him not to be able to see a damned thing. The imagination can take a bottom far beyond reality, and blindfolding him is one way to facilitate that journey.

Butterfly Boards. These are usually disposable foam or cork boards used for "butterflying." This play involves stretching the skin of the scrotum and pinning it to a board with sterile needles. This scene should not be done by an inexperienced person. Sterile technique is very important and infections of the scrotum can be very serious. If you are thinking about doing this, find an experienced player who knows this scene and get him or her to teach you. Book-learning is simply not sufficient for some things, and this is one of them.

Catheters. Sold in medical supply houses, these long plastic tubes are designed to be inserted into the urethra and up into the bladder in order to drain urine directly from the bladder. These must be medically sterile and cannot be reused for any reason (plastic/Teflon cannot be re-sterilized). There is not enough room to go into the use of catheters here, and it is also not something that would be easily learned from a book. I suggest finding a skilled catheter-play aficionado from whom to learn how to use these toys.

Anything inserted into the urethra creates a risk of infection, scarring, and/or tissue damage, and inserting things into the bladder increases the risk that any mishap might directly affect the kidneys. These things happen even in hospitals, even when done by professionals, so please, if you want to play with these toys, you owe it to yourself (and anyone else you play with) to learn from someone in your local BDSM community who has been doing it for a while and has a good track record for safety.

Clothespins. An old standby for cock and ball play is the spring-action wooden or plastic clothespin. From just a few to several dozen,

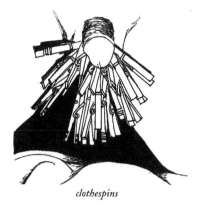

clothespins

these are great fun on the privates, particularly the scrotum and foreskin, and are unlikely to cause any damage. Clothespins that are too tight can be loosened by taking the clothespin apart and bending the wire spring so that the grip is looser when it is put back together.

Cock Rings. Cock rings are slender rings or straps that fit around the base of the cock, behind the balls. They can be made of many different materials, including metal, leather, and rubber, and can be a pre-made and pre-sized unbroken ring, an adjustable strap that can be held tightly in place with a fastener of some sort, or in some other adjustable configuration. Cock rings fit snugly enough around the base of the cock that they help keep blood in an erect cock from draining out, prolonging and possibly intensifying an erection.

When you choose a cock ring, bear in mind that sizing is important. One cock ring dealer suggests that you measure the circumference, or distance around, the base of your erect penis at the place where you will wear the cock ring. Divide by 3.1, and you have a reference number for an appropriate diameter for your cock ring. When in doubt, or between two sizes, however, choose the next higher available size of ring, since too tight can make for more serious problems than slightly loose.

Cock rings can sometimes be difficult to remove if the penis is hard or if one or more of the balls become swollen. This is particularly true of the one-piece, continuous cock rings, and especially the metal ones. The advantage of cock rings made out of rubber, leather, or fabric is that they can be cut off with a pair of heavy shears if need be. Any adjustable model can simply be made bigger for removal in case of an emergency. Should you get "stuck" in a cock ring and be unable to remove it, however, do not panic: just revisit the instructions on p. 31.

Combination Stretchers. These are cock rings with ball stretchers attached. They hold the cock erect while pushing the balls forward and away from the body.

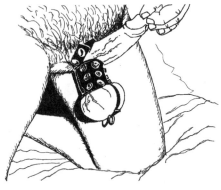

combinationstretcher

Elastic Bandages. Elastic bandages, such as ACE bandages, are nice, easy-to-use constriction devices for the cock and/or balls. They can also be used to keep the balls in place for other play. A nice combination is to wind an elastic bandage around the balls, then use a ball crusher or bar clamp on top to put pressure on the nuts. In a bandage, the testicles won't roll around, which tends to make them easier and safer to work with, whether for pressure or for impact play, such as tapping the nuts with a paddle or club.

Electrical Toys. There is a booming industry manufacturing cock and ball toys to be used in conjunction with the TENS (Transcutaneous Electrical Neural Stimulation) units and their BDSM-world equivalents. These units, which go by various names depending on the manufacturer, modify electrical current so that it can be hooked up to electrical stimulators on the skin, and the current used to produce physical sensation. The current is very low amperage but high voltage, and causes muscles to twitch as the device delivers pulses of electrical charge.

Special cock and ball play attachments, including conductive rubber catheters, cock rings, and sheaths, are available, but they tend to be

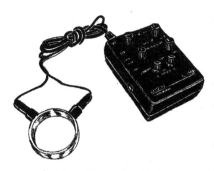

shock box with cock ring attachment

very expensive. Used in tandem with an electrical butt plug or electrically conductive dildo attached to the same shock box or similar device, a nice jolt can be delivered to the prostate gland from both sides. The sensation can be anywhere from tingly to painful to something resembling a continuous orgasm, depending on the intensity of the stimulation and the person's tolerance for those sensations. Electrical toys used for insertion should be considered "one-player" toys, since they are difficult to sterilize.

The latest electrical innovation I've seen is a cock and ball vise made to be attached to a shock box. Constructed of two layers of Plexiglas coated with conductive tape, this apparatus clamps the cock and balls flat, whereupon the conductive strips can deliver the desired electric sensations. Lots of fun, to be sure, but a major investment.

Another innovative electrical toy that some people like to use for cock and ball play comes directly from the pet store – a radio-controlled shock collar made for use in training dogs. This small device works much like a miniature cattle prod, except that it can be triggered using a battery-operated remote control. When this little number is strapped on, cock ring style, with the contact points under the scrotum, it can be very effective. As with all toys, however, this one is best tested on yourself before using it on anyone else, so you'll know just how intense it is. Bear in mind that not everyone has the same threshold of pain or taste in terms of types of stimulation, however, and be prepared to listen to feedback.

Hands. Hands are the cheapest and most effective cock and ball toys known to humankind. What you can do with your hands is far more effective than any other toy. Be creative and use your imagination.

I once watched in amazement at a scene involving only a top's hands, some lube, and a willing bottom in a masturbation scene that continued for over an hour. Each time the bottom was about to come, the top slapped the head of his cock and halted the stimulation. By the end of the scene, the bottom was screaming in his urgency to finally release the pent-up orgasm. When he finally did orgasm, you can bet it was a spiritual experience!

Ointments, Liniments, and Sports Rubs. Many over-the-counter ointments, liniments, and sports rubs are used to soothe sore muscles, and are well-known for the skin sensations they produce into the bargain. There are two primary types. Icy rubs, containing menthol, mint, camphor, eucalyptus, and similar oils, produce a cool tingling feeling. Hot rubs usually contain cinnamon oil, mustard oil, capsaicin (the chemical that makes hot chiles hot), or some combination. These oils irritate the skin and stimulate blood flow, causing a warming sensation and sometimes some actual heating of the skin itself.

Check the label to make sure that the compound you're using is safe for use on any part of the body. Capsaicin creams particularly can cause actual chemical burns, so be careful, and never get these creams or ointments in your (or anyone else's) eyes. Using latex exam gloves when you apply them, then taking the gloves off after you're done, is a great precaution to take, since you never know when you're going to forget what's on your hands and rub your eyes.

Because these compounds are oil-based, they do not wash off easily, which means that this is not a scene that is easy to stop suddenly. Using Ben Gay or other similar creams used to be a favorite locker room gag – Ben Gay in a jock strap turned a workout into a non-consensual scene that didn't necessarily end with a shower, since even hot water and lots of soap can't always remove all the residue of an oil. So don't use any of these compounds – Tiger Balm, Ben Gay, Icy Hot, or any other – as lube, within the urethra or rectum, or on any mucous membranes. They are not condom-friendly, they are hard to wash off or out of your body, and they may continue to burn for a long time, possibly far longer than you want them to. They may also cause chemical burns, particularly if there is any damage (hemorrhoids, fissures, cuts) in the tissues to which they are applied.

A water-soluble alternative, though it still isn't a good lube or lube additive, is toothpaste. It provides a nice tingle, and, since it is designed to be water-soluble, it washes off much more easily. Plus, you'll be minty fresh!

For instructions on dealing with a hot cream "overdose," see p. 31.

Parachutes. A conical leather collar or sheath that is fastened around the top of the balls, just below the penis. These often have attachment points or small chains already attached, either for the suspension of weights or for connecting a leash. The shape and chains give it a parachute appearance, with the "collar" portion being the parachute itself. I would caution users to not use extremely heavy weights with parachutes, as they may stretch and slip over one or both testicles. The resulting effect is much like being kicked in the groin!

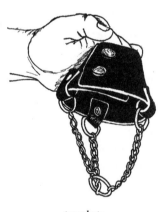

parachute

Rope. Rope is a basic tool for fun binding and stretching of the various dangling bits! Never underestimate the value of a good piece of rope. Keep bandage scissors or "EMT scissors" handy in case you need to do a quick release and don't have time to untie knots. *Jay Wiseman's*

Erotic Bondage Handbook is full of great advice about ropes, knotting, and techniques.

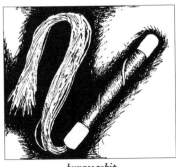

bungee whip

Rubber or "Bungee" Whips. These are small variations of a rubber flogger, and consist of a few dozen strands of rubber, very much like long rubber bands, attached to a stiff handle to facilitate easy use. The tips of these when spun or flailed against the skin, can feel very much like bee stings. The sound of a bungee whip spinning makes a very intimidating whistle, too.

Sheaths. Mostly made of leather, these resemble long ball stretchers but they are made to wrap the penis. They may be laced on, corset-style, or may have snaps or Velcro closures. A sheath prevents the surface of the penile shaft from being touched directly, while adding a sensation of constant constriction, and I have used them in a scene to keep a bottom from having too much access to his own penis. These are sometimes also called "cock corsets."

Steel Ball Harnesses. These resemble three steel cock rings welded together. They can be put on only when the penis is flaccid. The penis and balls go through the large ring, cock ring style. Then the penis is pushed through the top ring and the balls are manipulated one at a time through the base ring. I find I have to work fast when fitting these on someone, because erections happen very fast.

Studded Sheaths. These are very similar to the normal penis sheath, but they have the added feature of metal studs, or sometimes sharp prongs, on the inside. The points are usually not sharp enough to break the skin, but those with studs or prongs sharp enough to scratch should

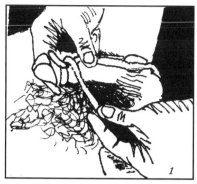
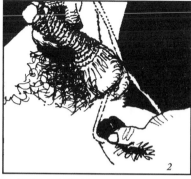

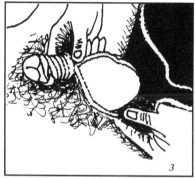
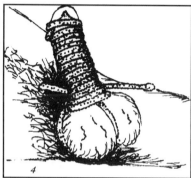

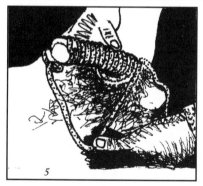

Starting with an 8' length of woven nylon rope, make a loop over the head of the cock. Pull about a foot of excess rope down along the underside of the shaft.

Begin wrapping the cock clockwise, in snug, even rows, with the rope along the shaft on the inside of the wrapping.

When the cock is wrapped to the base, wrap the rope around the base of the cock and scrotum, with the rope from the shaft separating the balls.

Continue wrapping around the balls, catching the ball-separating rope in the process. Then pull the ball-separating rope taut.

Tighten everything down and tie the ends together with a bow or other quick-release knot. Voila! a ball stretcher and cock sheath with nothing more than a piece of rope.

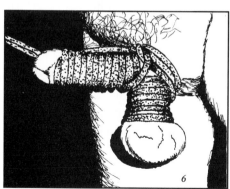

the toy box . 53

definitely be one-person toys. These are nice when working with a bottom who is becoming too excited too early. A simple squeeze of the sheath almost instantly reduces an erection to manageable proportions.

Thongs. Thongs, or laces, are long narrow pieces of leather or rubber. These are good basic tools for binding and stretching the various dangling bits. A good opportunity to practice your knot-tying and macramé. Keep bandage scissors handy in case you need to do a quick release and don't have time to untie knots.

Tweezers. Ever yanked out a pubic hair by accident, perhaps by catching it in your zipper? Then you already understand how effective it can be to pull out even a single hair by the roots. A good pair of tweezers – slant-tip tweezers are best, and be sure to either get them sharpened or buy a new pair regularly, as they become dull and will slip and break rather than grab and yank the hairs – is an invaluable and unassuming tool whose effect can be much greater than you might think.

Twitch. The twitch is a cast aluminum gadget used by vets on horses and mules. It is clamped on their lower lips to distract them while other, more delicate work is done on the animal. Twitches are sold in BDSM and leather shops as "ball crushers" for about five times the cost of a veterinary supply house. If you get one at the vet supply, be sure it is the screw

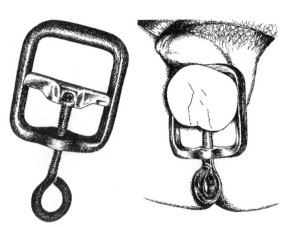

twitch (off and on)

type, not the older chair loop twitch. The twitch goes above the testicles themselves, and is clamped down so that it will not slip over the testicles and off of the scrotum. The twitch is *not* to be tightened down on the testes themselves, as this could cause serious damage. The weight of the twitch, and/or any weights you may choose to hang from it, is what does the "ball crushing," not the jaws of the twitch.

Urethral Sounds. These are medical devices used by urologists to clear the urinary passageways of strictures and blockages. They are steel rods, approximately eight or so inches in length, and come in an array of diameters. There are two primary types of urethral sounds, straight and curved (also called French sounds). Since these are used inside the urethra, they must be well sterilized before each use. Many professional piercing or tattooing parlors will autoclave your sounds for a nominal fee.

There is not enough room to go into the use of sounds here, and it is also not something that would be easily learned from a book. I suggest finding a skilled urethra-play aficionado from whom to learn how to use these toys. Anything inserted into the urethra creates a risk of infection, scarring, and/or tissue damage. These things happen even in hospitals and when done by professionals, so please, if you want to play with these toys, you owe it to yourself (and anyone else you play with) to learn from someone in your local BDSM community who has been doing it for a while and has a good track record for safety.

Vampire Gloves. These are thin leather "driving glove" type gloves to which small multi-pronged metal studs have been added so that the points protrude from the palm or the inside curves of the fingers. These can be used for stroking, gentle squeezing, or light slapping or tapping. Use caution, as these babies are sharp, and can easily pierce skin. If there is any question whether or not skin has been broken, it is best to regard vampire gloves as single-user toys, since they cannot be sterilized.

Wartenburg Wheels. Similar to tracing wheels used for sewing projects (in fact, you can use tracing wheels in the same ways), a Wartenburg wheel is a spur-like implement with a rotating disk of sharp little metal spikes at the end of a sticklike handle. Designed for neurological testing, a Wartenburg wheel will let you do some very intense neurological exploration of your own, producing sensations that range from the tingly to feeling almost as if one is being cut (depending on how much pressure is used), but with a very low risk of actually piercing or breaking the skin. If there is any question of whether the skin has been broken, however, the toy must be sterilized.

Pervertables

A "pervertable" is any common object not normally used for sexual purposes that can — with the creative insight only a sexually inventive mind can provide — be adapted for play. Two of the favorite shopping destinations of any budget-minded sexual explorer have long been hardware stores and kitchenware shops, and when you put on your kink-colored glasses, it's easy to see why. Here's a list of some of my favorite "pervertables" for cock and ball play. Some take a little modification, but most will work just fine right out of the package.

Basting Brushes. These come in a variety of styles with bristles of varying stiffness. These make great sensation toys, and a gentle brush across the right spot can whip up a bumper crop of goosbumps. Though paintbrushes can be used for the same things, basting brushes are preferable in one major respect — they are often dishwasher-safe, and if you happen to get any bodily fluids on them, running them through the dishwasher on the hottest setting is an excellent way to clean them up.

C-Clamps. No, not the big heavy-duty ones, the tiny kind used for clamping small woodworking projects and parts. Most measure about one and one-half to three inches, and work for any play involving clamps. Since these do screw completely closed, you should never tighten them down completely, as that would cause serious injury. Make sure that the flat portion of the clamp is free of metal burrs and sharp edges. You may need to use a fine grit sandpaper to smooth these down. The mere fact that these are hardware is both a turn-on and a threat to some people – a common reaction is "you're not going to put those on me, are you?" – and the psychological impact of using hardware in a scene can be very potent (as well as something to negotiate about beforehand!).

Dog Collars. Not as neckwear, but as accessories for genital bondage. Collars intended for small dogs can make perfect toys for genital bondage. You may need to punch a few more holes to ensure a tight fit, but most hardware stores will also stock leather punches so you can do this yourself. Can't you think of someone who'd look just stunning with a studded black leather poodle collar as a cock ring?

Egg Cutters or Scissors. These look a bit like scissors, except that where the blades should be, there is a metal ring. Squeeze the handles together, and two rows of curved metal points emerge from a channel in the ring. Placed over the top of a boiled egg, these neatly pierce the shell and open the top tidily for the eater. Many people have never seen one of these

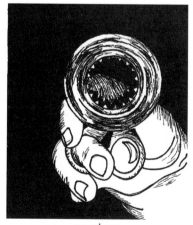

egg scissors

gadgets, so they make a good toy for those "do you know what this is?" guessing games. It won't take your playmate long to figure out that the ring can easily fit around something other than the top of a boiled egg! The points are usually not very sharp, but may easily be dulled down with a metal nail file to prevent any accidental puncture. Check before you play, and modify the toy if needed.

Fishing Sinkers and Net Weights. Lead sinkers and fishing net weights can be found in sporting-goods stores and in some larger hardware stores that carry sporting equipment. You can find sinkers and net weights in a variety of weights, but I find that sinkers for open-water fishing, usually four or five ounces in weight, are a good versatile size. These can be attached to any kind of ball stretcher, though I do not recommend using very much weight with a parachute, as parachutes can stretch and may slip off painfully when weighted. As an added touch, you can paint or rubber-coat lead weights to give them a more attractive finish and to minimize contact with the lead surface.

Hamburger and Meatball Presses. Who knew you could use these on other kinds of meat? These are great sensation toys, particularly the metal ones… and particularly when they're cold (cold water or an ice bucket is a good way to chill things down). Used for gentle squeezing, these are great things to try if you're feeling adventurous. Never close them completely, though, as this could cause serious damage.

Miniature Spatulas. Mini versions of large rubber spatulas make great slappers for cock and ball play. The tips are often very flexible and have just enough give so that they deliver a nice sting. Try yours on the inside of your elbow or thigh first to get an idea of just how intense the sting tends to be.

Mouse and Rat Traps. This is one "pervertable" you should never use out of the box without modifying it first. There are too many sharp edges on the trigger pads. However, with little effort, you can remove the trigger altogether, and, with some fine-grit sandpaper, round off the wooden corners and sand everything down in order to prevent splinters. When using mouse or rat traps, do not release the springs full force on any part of anyone's body – not a finger, and definitely not someone's genitals. However, if applied slowly on the foreskin or scrotum (avoid pinching the testicle), the springs are not strong enough to do damage, and the visual effect can be stunning and intimidating. The sound of the trap being snapped in midair is also a very effective psychological tool.

Mushroom Brushes. These little brushes have moderately soft bristles and are great for focusing sensation on a man's "mushroom" or balls. These brushes often feel tickly at first, and quite tolerable, but the sensation will become more intense as the area becomes more sensitized. A warning: these are very soft, but repeated friction can cause friction burns or abrasions. Do keep in mind that when someone is aroused, the line between pain and pleasure can become very blurry indeed. If things start to look a little too red, or if the skin looks traumatized, it's probably best to stop and try a different type of sensation.

Pulleys, Blocks and Tackle. Many hardware stores now carry smaller versions of the traditional block and tackle. These devices are intended for lifting small amounts of weight and often have a ratchet brake system which prevents the object being lifted from falling down until it is released. I keep a pair of these in my toy box. Whenever I need to stretch or suspend a partner's naughty bits, these can come in very handy. The ratchets add a nice sound effect, too.

Spring or "Pony" Clamps. These are the larger metal clamps with rubber handles and rubber or vinyl-covered tips. The big ones are too strong for use in cock and ball play, but some of the small ones have little more bite than clothespins and can be fun toys. Definitely test these before you buy. The skin between thumb and forefinger works well. It is almost as soft as scrotal skin and is quite sensitive, so if you can't stand it "up North," you definitely won't like it "down South." If in doubt, err on the side of caution.

A Final Word About Toys

Every day, some twisted genius comes up with a new plaything to be used in conjunction with the family jewels, so trying to make a truly complete compendium would be impossible. The great thing about cock and ball toys in general is that they are usually either fairly reasonable in price, or else they are often easier to make than you might think. If there's some item you've seen in a BDSM shop that really caught your eye, but was unaffordable, chances are that you can figure out how to make a reasonable facsimile yourself for much less. Yours may not be as pretty or shiny, but the effect will be just as good!

Keep in mind, too, that you don't need a whole toy chest full of toys to have fun. While having fun and esoteric toys is enjoyable, owning just the ones that work for you and/or your playmates is certainly enough to fill the bill. There's no need to go overboard, particularly if it'd do violence to your financial bottom line. Hands, as you may recall, are a fine toychest all by themselves, and they're available absolutely free.

I am a firm believer in the practice of trying out all toys on myself before I try them on someone else. Without a test-drive, it's hard to know what the range of sensations produced by any given toy might be like. It's also sensible to remember that your limits and thresholds are not going to be the same as the next person's. You may feel that a particular clamp is quite lightweight, but a playmate may have a much lower threshold of pain when it comes to clamps and clips. For him, the clamp you barely felt could be excruciating. Start small and light, then work your way up to heavier stimulation: doing it the other way around will end a scene before it has a chance to begin.

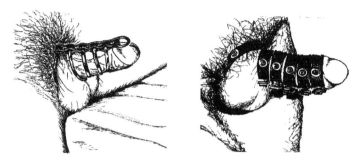

some specialty toys: "five gates of hell," in steel and leather

4.

Soup to Nuts:

CBT

Techniques

and "Recipes"

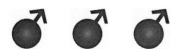

Let's assume the stage is set. You're rarin' to go, you have a play partner or two, and of course, you have the most important elements of all, cocks and balls. You've got some toys you'd like to play with, too, and a pretty good idea of the kinds of things you'd like to try. You've negotiated things with your playmate(s), settled on a safeword… so now what?

How do you put it into practice, and what can you expect when you do?

The sets of instructions and short stories that follow are intended to help you as you take that next step. Like a good teaching cookbook, equipment and techniques are presented first, with a little discussion of how the various types of cock and ball play enacted in each story are done, what to watch out for, and so on. The "In Context" vignettes that follow are a bit like recipes, showing you how those techniques might work within scenes. Unlike a recipe, though, the descriptions of scenes are not intended as step-by-step instructions for what you (or your partner(s) in any scene) should do. They're intended as illustrations, to give you some context, show you how the techniques might play out in practice, and, I hope, to arouse you sufficiently to try some of the techniques yourself.

Before you try any of these techniques on another person, however, I strongly suggest that you try them on yourself. This is easy enough to do, as long as you're male. For women, transgendered folk, and other people who may not have the requisite configuration of external genitalia to practice on, on the other hand, it poses a little bit of a problem. What's an enterprising, but non-cock-and-ball-owning, person to do?

Well, basically, you do the same thing as a person with his own set of goodies to practice on would do, but you do it with a friend, and you do it much more carefully. Whenever you're doing something to another person's body, the thing to do is to work slowly and carefully, making sure that you pay close attention to their reactions and asking for their detailed feedback.

You may also want to make some contacts in your local BDSM community and arrange to observe some cock and ball play sessions between experienced players, or to have a knowledgeable top who is well-versed in this kind of play give you some one-on-one tutoring. This kind of learning scene is not very hard to negotiate. Most people, when asked to share their knowledge and experience, take it as a compliment. Even if you are unsuccessful in persuading an experienced cock and ball player to give you private lessons, you will undoubtedly find one who will at least share some hints and tips. A side advantage of a session with an experienced player is the benefit of getting to see, and perhaps try out, items from their toybox. There are few things as discouraging as bringing home an expensive new cock and ball toy and finding out either you or your partner just doesn't like it. Since most leather shops take a dim view of returned merchandise, especially if it's used, getting a chance to test drive someone else's toys can be really helpful. Don't forget to thank your benefactor!

It's not impossible for someone who doesn't have a cock and balls to learn cock and ball play, and even to become extremely good at it – but it does take care, common sense, and empathy, the same things that it takes for anyone to learn how to engage in this kind of play with expertise and just the right blend of sadism, common sense, delight, sensuality, and compassion.

Here are some tips to help make sure your learning curve is a smooth one. These hold no matter whether you try things out on yourself first or not, whether you have a penis and balls or not. Treat each new partner as if he were your first, and remember that everyone is different, which means that we have to learn how each individual person will respond to the kinds of stimulation used in cock and ball play.

- Keep communication flowing. Make sure you ask how things feel as you go along.

- Ask about intensity. Is it too much, or not enough? What should be different?

- Ask about how different things feel: if, for instance, you are squeezing someone's balls, ask how it feels if you squeeze them in different ways and with differing degrees and directions of force. Sometimes differences that seem subtle to you can feel major to someone else.

- Whenever you are hitting or flogging someone's cock or balls, hold the bottom's genitals in your hand and make sure you hit your hand as well as you strike the bottom's body. This will give you a good indication of how hard you are hitting.

- Watch for nonverbal reactions. Facial expressions, winces or flinches, tensing of muscles in the face or torso, clenched hands, gasps, holding the breath, and other nonverbal signs can be very valuable indicators of how someone is feeling or processing stimulation.

- Above all, pay attention. If you are paying close attention to your play partners as people, and not just as cocks and balls, you will probably be fine.

Just A Little Handiwork

Equipment

Hands

Water-based personal lubricant

(Wartenburg wheel – optional)

Techniques

Stroking, tugging, caressing, squeezing, and general manual stimulation of the penis and scrotum – essentially, a handjob, which is best performed by experimenting with strokes and squeezes and figuring out what seems to work best on your individual partner.

Using water-based personal *lube* is a wonderful adjunct to almost any genital sex, and particularly for handjobs and masturbation. If the lube you're using starts to dry out, either apply more lube or use a bit of warm water to reactivate the lubrication. If you are doing a cock and ball play scene only, and are not engaging in any genital sex (oral-genital, anal-genital, or genital-genital contact), however, you can feel free to use an oil-based lubricant such as massage oil, lotion, cold cream, etc., if that is what you prefer. For health reasons and for safer sex reasons (oil can cause problems inside the body, and disintegrates latex), however, do not use oil-based lubricants if you are going to have any sort of genital sexual contact during or following play.

Using a *Wartenburg wheel* on the genitals takes some care. Use a light touch unless you are very sure that your play partner is up for more – those pin-like spines are sharp! Do not attempt to use the Wartenburg wheel to puncture the skin, that's not what it's for. Just glide the wheel over the skin, and watch the incredible response.

In Context

Some of the hottest cock and ball scenes I've ever seen involved little more than a pair of hands, and every time I remember the closing night party at the Leatherfest, I still find myself aroused.

As a gay man, I might've thought that watching a straight couple play would seem a little uninteresting, but these two were an incredible exception. In their mid-thirties, and pleasing to the eye, they chose a small bondage table near the corner of the dungeon as the setting for their scene. By their looks, I almost assumed they were just tourists who wandered into something they had only read about in magazines, but boy, did they ever prove that impression wrong.

He stripped out of his chinos and golf shirt, while she opened the small black bag she carried. When he was completely naked, she pointed to the table. He dutifully climbed on and lay flat on his back. She pulled out a few short lengths of thick nylon rope and deftly tied his hands and feet to the eyelets at the corners of the table. I have to admit he looked a lot better buck naked and spread-eagled. She smiled at me with a knowing twinkle, as if to say, "come on over and watch, if you'd like." I took the invitation.

Next, she snapped on a pair of latex surgical gloves like she was a surgeon preparing for an operation, and her purposeful expression got my full attention. In one move, she had a simple adjustable leather cock ring fastened securely around the base of her partner's cock and balls, and as they began to engorge with blood, I moved a little closer to get a better look at what was promising to be a very nice cock. Last, but not least, she took out a bottle of lube, squirting some into her hand and letting the heat of her palm warm it up.

Then, slowly and deliberately, she began to smear the lubricant around the head of his cock. Starting at the tip and moving very slowly down in lazy circles, she smeared the clear lube along the entire length of his now rigid penis. Once it was coated with the glistening gel, she held the base with one hand and slowly traced the length of his dick with her forefinger, smearing lube as she went. When I say she did this slowly, I mean she did it *excruciatingly* slowly, and every second of the way she watched his face and the marvelous expressions he made.

When she had finally reached the tip again, she took his cock between her thumb and forefinger and started stroking back down, even slower than before. This time he began to make small breathy gasps. By this time, I was transfixed. I could hear him gasp as her fingers ran over each vein of his rock hard cock. Reaching the base of his cock, she removed her hand and started back at the tip, this time with three fingers, slowly moving down again. She kept this up until she was using her whole hand, encircling his throbbing cock and slowly stroking it, always in a downward motion. I had no concept of how much time had passed, but when I took my mind off the scene for only a few seconds, I realized that the CD that was playing from a nearby boom box was already half over.

As she sped up her actions, she continued her downward strokes. They were almost like thrusts, her fist wrapping his cock and pushing down toward the base in long sweeps.

Within a few minutes she was working full speed, slamming her fist over his cock, ramming toward the base and then releasing just before reaching his abdomen, and he was groaning, deep and throaty. There was just no way she could keep that sort of treatment up much longer without his cock exploding. I was sure he was just about to come – and probably would've, but instead, she stopped.

Breathless, he managed to let out a rattling groan. Apparently, his exquisite torture for the evening was to be brought to the brink of ejaculation and then left helpless on the edge. I could not take my eyes off of them. She apparently knew his body so well that she could anticipate his orgasm, and stop just prior to that point of no return. To help him calm back down, she whipped out a Wartenburg wheel and slowly ran it along the length of his penis. In his state of hypersensitivity, this made him howl like an animal, and his cock ceased its swelling, at least temporarily. But soon she began the whole process over again, taking him right to the edge of his orgasm, then bringing him back.

This wild scene lasted well over two hours before she finally stroked him to a full ejaculation, a tremendous orgasm in which he shot a good three feet straight into the air, probably due to all the tremendous tension and yearning he was enduring at her hands. Only after he was spent did the domme again acknowledge my presence, smiling knowingly and glancing toward my crotch. I know the room was too dimly lit for her to have seen the dark wet spot on the front of my black jeans, but I'm sure she knew by my expression that it had been good for me too!

All Pins, No Needles

Equipment
Wooden or plastic spring-action clothespins

Techniques
When placing a *clothespin* on a loose bit of skin, first pinch the skin into a suitable fold with your fingers. Bear in mind that letting the jaws of a clothespin close gently feels different from simply letting them snap into place. The same is true of how you take them off. Much like removing a Band-Aid, ripping them off feels quite different from taking them off slowly. Experiment! You may be surprised at the range of nuance you can get from such a simple toy.

The sensation produced by clothespins or any other clips or clamps is intense at first, but fades after a few minutes as the blood supply gets cut off in the clamped tissue. Don't forget, though, that when you take the clothespin off and that blood comes rushing back, the sensation will come rushing back right along with it – a clothespin bites twice!

Because clothespins and other clips and clamps do cut off the blood supply to the clamped skin after a while, don't leave them on for extended periods of time, particularly if you have many of them on. Thirty minutes is about the maximum length of time you should leave clothespins on someone.

In Context

You and your sweetie have gone off camping – the hill country is just gorgeous this time of year, and you know the perfect remote spot miles away from pretty much anything. You know the chances of anyone dropping by are next to nil, so you decide to try a little outdoor play. Your materials are limited, but your girlfriend has a wicked grin on her face: she brought along a small toy bag, just in case.

After a short discussion, consisting mainly of her whispering wonderful, wicked ideas in your ears, you readily agree to become the object of her desire. She begins by telling you to strip naked except for your hiking boots. The ground is rocky, and she doesn't want you to injure your feet. Besides, this is Texas, and you never know when you might step on a bed of fire ants!

So you leave your boots on, but take off everything else, exposed to the sky, the sun, and your partner's appraising glance. She tosses a blanket on the ground, and then orders you to kneel. You bow your head obediently and await further instructions, since she hasn't told you how or where. She breaks a twig from a nearby willow tree and uses it to coax your hands behind your back. *Thwack!* A sharp sting to your shoulders gets the point across. She wants your ass in the air, clearly, so you lean over and nestle your head in your hands, your tush raised for her amusement. Wave after wave of warm sensation sweeps over you, making the base of your balls tingle, with each swat of the willow branch across your butt. After a few dozen strokes, she allows you to once again kneel upright. Your ass stings, almost a buzzing sensation, as it rests against the heels of your hiking boots.

Then your eyelids snap wide open at the sound of the contents of that toybag being dumped onto the blanket. It's clothespins, about fifty of them! This is going to be some intense fun. She moves a campstool into position several feet in front of you and sits down. She orders you to crawl to her and show your appreciation for what she has done and is about to do, and you do so dutifully, head bowed. Submissively, you start to lick her boots as a gesture of your appreciation, eagerly cleaning every trace of the hot 'n' dusty trail from the well-worn leather with your tongue.

Your Mistress is merciful, lucky for you, and she soon decides to reward your good behavior, slipping off the campstool and telling you to sit. She has you sit on the stool, and she kneels between your legs, reaching out to grab your half-erect cock with a firm grip. Stroking it a few times, she lifts it to get better access to your balls, holding your cock out of the way as she picks up that thin willow branch again and playfully teases the loose skin of your scrotum to watch your reaction.

Shortly, she puts down the stick and pinches a bit of scrotum skin just at the base of your cock, scrutinizing your face as she applies the pressure. You smile, trying to hide the half-pained expression you instinctively want to make. She winks at you and applies more pressure. It instantly becomes a game: how long will you continue smiling and not show any pain, and how long can she continue to up the ante before you do?

With a satisfied, teasing smile, she assures herself that you understand the rules, the body language between the two of you saying more than words could. Then she takes a clothespin and puts it on the same spot she was pinching. She toys with it a bit before adding another snug little clamp just next to it, gathering another small fold of scrotum skin and giving it a pinch before she lets the clothespin take over for her fingertips. You feel the mild aching of the pinched skin, but know that it won't last long: once the blood has been cut off for a few minutes, the nerves will stop sending their message to the brain and a heavy numbness will settle in. You continue to force a smile as she adds clothespin after clothespin, making a neat row around the base of your scrotum. Your balls look like the center of a daisy, with clothespin petals extending in all directions!

She adds another row next to the first, and follows that with another, concentric circles of clothespins slowly covering the entire scrotal sac. What once were nice fleshy dangling balls now look like a wooden porcupine, and the opiates triggered deep within your brain in response to the continued pain of the pins puts a broad – and very genuine – grin across your face. You don't have to try to smile now. It feels *good*.

She sees this and starts to laugh, knowing that the effects of her work on your scrotum are already metamorphosing from pain into pleasure. With a stroke of the willow switch across your thighs, she orders you to stand up. You get to your feet carefully, hoping the pins won't pinch any worse, but she has other plans for you, and promptly whacks you across the ass and orders you to move. The pins rattle like castanets as you take your first few tentative steps. The weight on your balls is an amazing feeling, but before you can savor it she has you running back and forth across the campsite, taunting you with that willow switch, telling you to lift your feet like a show pony to make those clothespins rattle all the more.

You are laughing and wincing and panting by the time she brings you to a halt. She kneels and rattles your clothespin-studded scrotum a few times, running her finger along the clothespins like dragging a stick along a picket fence, then looks up and gives you the bad news: they have to come off. And you know that when those pins come off, the nerve endings will explode into life as the blood returns, firing off an extraordinary fusillade of sensation.

With measured moves, she slowly pulls off the first pin. Then another, and another. Soon you are spouting obscenities. This is just what she wants. *Snap! Snap!* She continues, accelerating the pace, the pain from each pin flowing through you and colliding with the pain from the next, until there is only one pin left. Delicately, she puts her fingers on it, then looks up at you with a meaningful, totally wicked smile. She doesn't move to take it off of you. Clearly, she's expecting you to back away from her and basically pull it off yourself – a lovely and twisted little flourish.

Snap! You fall to your knees and she takes you in her arms, lowering the both of you to the ground. As you lay back against the blanket, you cannot help giggling, floating on a delicious combination of endorphins, sunshine, and attention from the woman you love. Gazing up at the sky, you feel the breeze on your hypersensitive scrotum, even a slight movement of air capable of sending shivers up and down your spine. Ain't nature grand?

Blue Balls

Equipment
Rubber-tailed "bungee" whip
Ball stretcher
(Shoe polish – optional)

Technique
Using any implement to strike or whip someone's cock and/or balls is something to be approached with a bit of care. Not only are the cock and balls very sensitive, but thresholds of pain vary widely from person to person. *"Bungee" whips (or floggers),* with their thin rubber tails, can pack a serious sting, so start slowly and work your way up. Your own hand can be a good gauge: hold your partner's cock/balls in your hand

as you work with the flogger or whip, and make sure to hit your hand as you hit your partner. That way you get a very precise idea of how hard you're hitting. When you combine the knowledge of how hard you're hitting with the reactions you get from your partner, you can develop a very acute awareness of exactly how to use your tools to produce the desired effect.

Experiment with different strokes with the flogger. Flogger tails can be tickled or draped against the skin, shaken so that just the tips brush against the flesh, flicked at a person in much the same way that a horse flicks its tail, and so on. Even the strokes used for more intense blows can be enormously varied: overhand, underhand, sidearm, figure-eight. If you are new to using whips and floggers, or simply have a new one you're not used to yet, practice on a pillow first until you get a feel for the implement and know how to aim it with a reasonable degree of accuracy. You want to avoid hitting things other than your intended target, obviously, both for safety's sake and to concentrate the effect.

When it comes to *ball stretchers*, choose one that the intended wearer can comfortably accommodate. This will probably mean choosing a smaller one over a larger one at first. You can always work your way up. Even shorter, smaller ones have a decided effect on the wearer, so don't get something that's too big to be worn simply because you think a shorter ball stretcher won't provide the desired effect: it will.

In Context

Cock and ball play is delightful not only for the reactions your "boys" have to the treatment you give them, but because of the reactions you get from other people who may be watching. This weekend, there's a Club run – your local men's BDSM organization, camping out and hanging out on acres of private, wooded space, with plenty of well-outfitted playspaces to share and enjoy. It's a perfect opportunity to give your best "boy" and a hopeful new recruit a chance to strut their stuff, and for all of you to watch other folks' reactions to the trouble you get up to.

Your "boys" meet you before lunch in the main play area of the run compound. Here, under the shady canopy of a big tent, are a variety of tables and crosses standing ready for use. Gazing across the space, you turn to your playmates and order both lads to strip to their boots. Eagerly they pull off their clothes, and you already sense a little bit of competition between them. Your 'boy' knows he comes first in your heart, and that no one else can replace him, but he still likes to vie for your attention, and he always has been a bit of a show-off.

When both men are stripped and ready, you stand them back to back. Using a couple of leather belts, you strap them together around the chest and waist, a lovely and effective form of bondage that lets each man feel, quite intimately, the reactions of the other one even though they can't see each other. There is a rack nearby with a hanging chain. You order them to walk to it – which they do pretty awkwardly, and you almost burst out laughing watching them – and stand directly under the chain. When they have arrived, you take a spreader bar and attach it to the two hanging chains like a trapeze, dangling it just within reach above their heads.

"Grab that bar, boys," you say, and they do, reaching up and spreadeagling themselves for your pleasure. You're now free to open up your toy bag and get down to work, and you do, thinking about the fact that both men have been telling you for days just how eager they have been to play with you now.

After choosing the implement you want, you straighten up and withdraw a long, slender object from your shirt pocket and place it between your lips. Thoughtfully, you light the cigar, and puff on it to get it going. The taste is pleasant, the look is authoritarian, and occasionally the hot ash from the tip comes in handy in a scene. You blow a wisp of cool blue smoke into your boy's face. He eagerly sucks up the vapor. Then you walk to the other side and do the same to your new recruit. He blinks and tries to suck up some of the smoke, but it just isn't his scene. You decide not to press the issue, especially since he is new, and he might not be able to tolerate cigar smoke. An asthma attack would be dramatic, yes, but not quite the kind of dramatic you're looking for. Verbal action seems like the way to go.

Playing on the images that cigar generates in your mind, you decide to put on your Marine drill sergeant persona, eyeing your newer playmate with a cool, appraising eye. "You ever had your balls whipped, boy?" you bark.

"No sir," he answers respectfully.

"What did you say, boy?"

"I said, no sir, sir," he replies, louder this time. He is very distinct and loud, but you decide to push it further so he'll catch on completely to your game.

"I can't hear you, boy!" you snap, shouting like a seasoned leatherneck.

He gets it and smiles, then shouts back." I SAID NO SIR, SIR! I HAVE NEVER HAD MY BALLS WHIPPED, SIR!"

"Well, you got quite a treat coming to you, boy."

"THANK YOU, SIR. I AM SURE I WILL LIKE IT, SIR."

"I'm sure you will, too," you sigh menacingly under your breath, walking back to your "boy" and reaching down to grab his cock and balls.

"Now, my boy has had his balls whipped before, and he told me it was a little bit of heaven, didn't you, boy?"

Your boy smiles and you see that mischievous twinkle in his eye. "YES SIR!" he shouts, bright and cheerful. You pull his cock and balls away from his body until he is standing on tiptoe, his face starting to twist in pain.

"Yes sir *what*?" you taunt, knowing how much he loves the military-style order-giving, the shouting back and forth.

"YES SIR, A LITTLE BIT OF HEAVEN, SIR," he barks back as his nipples and cock start to harden. You keep up the drill sergeant routine for a few more minutes, pacing around the two naked men, watching their reactions. But why keep them waiting any longer? Pulling out the toy you'd chosen earlier, a flogger made of rubber strands similar to rubber bands, you give it a whirl near your "boy's" face. It whistles as the tails slice through the air, and you continue spinning it, listening to the warbling noise as the rubber strands break the air. Slowly, slowly, you move it down toward his half-erect cock, moving it gradually closer until the tips of the rubber tails graze the head of his cock. He winces and tries to pull away, but when he backs up he is locked by the boy strapped to his back, and you grin at him as he realizes he's stuck.

Now it's time to work his nuts. You lift his cock out of the way and begin a slow flogging of his balls. Starting with light sweeps, only gradually increasing the force of the strokes, you watch his face for reactions. Wincing and groaning are signs he is taking it well. You've been playing with him for quite a while and know his body language, but even so you watch him carefully. If you see an unfamiliar expression, or some sign of panic, you can ease off and keep the scene going longer. In a few minutes he is writhing and twisting, occasionally pulling his feet up off the floor. The combination of your whipping his balls and massaging the head of his cock while you hold it out of the way is sending him over the top.

Of course, it won't do to give one "boy" all the attention and leave the other one hanging. So you give your first panting victim a little while to catch his breath while you turn your attentions to the new kid in town. He gets the same treatment, but since he is new, you don't have such an intimate knowledge of his body language. To assure that you will be able to know his status, you encourage him to keep giving you feedback – a drill sergeant is perfectly able to command his charges to report on how each and every stroke feels. The necessity of responding keeps his attention focused on what's happening, and keeps you up-to-date on how he's doing, too. Besides which, it's hot... and as long as he continues with the "thank you sir, may I have another, sir," routine, there's little question of whether he's doing okay. You don't stop working him over until his dick begins to drip precum. You don't actually want him to orgasm, just to keep him excited and stimulated and waiting for what will happen next.

Now it's time to go back where you started, working over your longtime playmate with more of the same. He gets into the spirit of the scene by barking back the same words, "Thank you, sir! May I have another, sir!" and it becomes a noisy event, but one full of energy and enthusiasm. Soon both boys are dripping with sweat, vibrating from the sensations, and in need of a rest. So you decide to give them a rest – but not too much of one.

"ATTEN-SHUN!" you shout, and almost laugh when they instantly drop their hands to their sides and snap upright, their bodies as stiff as their cocks. "You boys have been doin' real good," you continue. "So I'm going to give you a little break. We're gonna take a walk around, stretch your legs, but just so everyone here knows what part of your scrawny anatomy I've been working on, I'm gonna give you something to wear."

You are already opening your bag. You've prepared for this in advance, and have a bottle of liquid shoe polish at the ready – in a distinguished and appropriately military shade of vivid navy blue. After showing your playmates the bottle, you pop off the cap and grab one man's aching balls. He winces, but keeps his eyes on you as you move the dauber over the wrinkled skin of his balls, leaving a deep blue trail. With just a few strokes, his balls are an impressive blue, so you move to your other victim and paint his as well. After you give the shoe polish a few minutes to dry, you take out a pair of heavy leather ball stretchers and collar their scrotums in the close-fitting leather, making sure the D-rings attached to them are front and center.

After removing the belts from around the men's chests and waists, you ready them for a little promenade, hands cuffed behind their backs, dog leashes clipped to those D-rings. For the next half-hour, you parade these two obedient and delighted boys around the grounds while you visit with friends and observe the other goings-on, and when the bright midday sun hits that navy blue shoe polish, everyone who wants to look will have an excellent idea of what's been going on. By the time you let them hit the showers to wash off the shoe polish, most of it will have been sweated away – but though the color will wear off, the memories of a fabulous scene, with the best possible kind of blue balls, will linger for a long, long time.

Double Your Pleasure

Equipment
Rope

Ratchet and pulley set

Bamboo skewers

Rubber "bungee" whip (see preceding chapter)

Techniques
When considering what kind of *rope* to use for genital bondage, you will want to carefully consider issues of rope thickness and abrasiveness. Some types of rope, particularly jute, are very scratchy and could cause unwanted abrasions. Slender, smooth-surfaced woven nylon cord is available at sporting goods and marine supply stores. Even cotton clothesline would be appropriate for this kind of play. Likewise, thickness matters. A rope that is too thick will be difficult to wrap and tie, first of

all, plus it won't allow you to wrap more than a few times around a man's penis or balls, leaving you with a distinct possibility that one or more of the turns of the rope might slip off. Since this could cause unplanned pain and even tissue damage, it's better to get a thinner rope that can fit more securely.

Keep in mind that the load, or amount of weight, you will expect your rope to bear. Most cock and ball play will not put a very substantial load on a rope, but if there is any doubt, check the tensile strength of the rope before you use it for play.

Pulleys and ratchet sets are something to experiment with well in advance of a scene. You should be familiar with how to set them up, how to thread the ropes through them, and how the planned setup will work.

You need to make sure that you have adequate attachment points – S-hooks or O-rings countersunk into suitable surfaces, like doorways or support beams, or other similarly sturdy attachment points – and that they are anchored and sturdy. Even though you are unlikely, when doing cock and ball play, to put a huge amount of weight or stress on your ropes and pulleys, you still need to make sure that nothing is fragile, loose, or likely to give way. Attachment points for any bondage or bondage apparatus, generally speaking, should be able to support at least twice as much strain as you plan to put on them, since torque can add exponentially to the stress on an attachment point or apparatus.

The narrow, somewhat flexible shafts of *bamboo skewers* can be used for many things, but they are particularly effective as slappers, used to strike the cock or balls. One way to do this is to hold the pointed end securely in your dominant hand (this helps ensure your aim) and hold the shaft of the skewer parallel to and about a quarter of an inch or so away from the area you want to strike. Use your index finger on the other hand to bend the skewer backwards slightly, then let it snap forward, striking the target area. You can also simply strike with the skewer as if it were a drumstick. Make sure not to use the pointed ends to hit with, as they are very sharp!

Be aware that sometimes bamboo skewers can be rough, and may be slightly splintery. Giving them a good rubbing with a layer or two of paper towel, or with a piece of slightly rough cloth (the leg of your jeans is good) will help remove any splinters that could unintentionally injure your partner(s).

In Context

Once in a while I get a chance to really show off and let the exhibitionist in me out to play. I'm not the type of person who likes to parade around naked, or have sex while others watch. I haven't got the body or the ego for that. No, I'm much more like a magician out to wow the crowds with his latest tricks.

It was one of those nights when I just couldn't help myself. I had been part of a seminar on cock and ball play, and afterward I attended a party in honor of the presenters. Before I could even get a cup of coffee, I was approached by a dominatrix who asked if I would demonstrate a few of my techniques on two of her male subs. I, of course, was already prepared with a small bag of tricks, and readily agreed.

Both young men were slim, attractive, and heterosexual, and more than a little nervous at the prospect of a man working on their private parts. I spoke for a few moments with both of them and assured them that I would do nothing to embarrass them in front of their Mistress, and that as far as I was concerned, anything beyond the arranged cock and ball play was out of the question. They gave a collective sigh of relief and stripped off their clothes, and we all moved into our host's garage, where a large wooden swing-set frame, swings removed, provided an ideal frame for bondage.

I had each of the submissives stand with his back to one of the uprights, then bound their hands behind their backs, behind the posts.

They certainly weren't going to go anywhere, but just to steady them, I tied an additional rope harness around each man's chest. With two naked men facing each other across a six or seven-foot expanse, I took a few moments to do the geometry and started to work on my setup.

I took two pulleys from my play bag and attached them with snap hooks to the eyelets where the swings once hung. The two boys watched intently, but gave no signs of arousal yet. So I took a couple of long pieces of rope from my bag and went to work on their cocks, deftly wrapping rope harnesses that cinched round the base of the cock and balls, then wrapped a few turns of rope around their upper scrotums to serve as ball stretchers, pushing their testicles away from their bodies. After making a knot to secure these impromptu ball stretchers, I took the remaining rope and threaded it through the pulleys. When I pulled on the ropes at the center of the swing set, each submissive's balls pulled up and away from his body, making him groan with pleasure. It was almost like playing the bells, gently tugging on a rope to hear the peal of sound that resulted.

Then I tied the ropes together, effectively tying one man's balls to the other's. After tying the ropes together, I hung a small dumbbell weight from the ends. Now it was the weight that was doing the work, and when I gently swung it back and forth, it alternately pulled one boy's balls and then the other, a swinging pendulum of painful pleasure.

Seeing that their cocks were growing by the minute, I decided to take two additional pieces of rope and wind them around their shafts, sheathing each one in tight coils of rope. Now they were rock hard and groaning in stereo. Their Mistress walked behind them and started whispering in their ears. I have no idea what she said, but whatever it was, it made their already turgid cocks strain at their rope bonds.

With them all tied up with no place to go, I could take my time, tending first to one of the lads, then the other. Using a small bamboo skewer, I snapped it against their bulging scrotums, eliciting grunts of pain and pleasure. After a few minutes, I switched to using my favorite bungee whip on them, stinging their balls with the thin rubber strands. Soon, their mistress decided that the two submissives were being far too noisy for their own good. With a wicked grin, she pulled a pair of large rubber dildos from her toybag and put one in each lad's mouth, effectively muffling the groans that continued unabated as I continued to torture the two men's shining red balls until they were dancing on tiptoe.

When I finally decided to begin bringing the scene to a close, I first removed the weight from the tied-together rope ends, then untied the ropes and pulled them free from the pulleys. Untying the knots that held the cock and ball harnesses on, I pulled the ropes gently, watching the men's balls do an exquisitely sensitive little dance as the rope that had been stretching their scrotums unspooled from around them. They accompanied their own dancing testicles with a little chorus of heartfelt groaning – nothing feels quite like being released from genital bondage after a really good scene.

Once they had been released from their bonds, the men's Mistress had them thank me properly by kissing my boots. I was gratified to see what a lovely bridge between worlds a little cock and ball play can be – two straight boys, once so shy about playing with a gay topman, hugged my legs and kissed my boots repeatedly in gratitude. I am given to understand that later on, they showed their gratitude to their Mistress as well, and provided for her the kind of heartfelt thank-you that I know she thoroughly enjoyed.

Yippee Tie 'Em Up!

Equipment

Rope

Knife

Velcro

Techniques

When selecting *rope*, please refer to the guidelines given previously on page 80. While individual bondage techniques are a matter of taste, and there are probably an infinite number of ways to put someone into body or genital bondage, remember that all bondage should be done safely. I recommend *Jay Wiseman's Erotic Bondage Handbook* as an excellent overview of technique and safety.

One thing you will want to bear in mind for a scene like the one described below is that different types of rope are suited to different types of use. For restraining someone's arms and legs, you may wish a different type of rope than you would use for genital bondage. Consider the types of bondage you are planning to do in a scene before selecting your rope: the right tool for the job is important and will make the experience better for everyone.

Knife play can be a powerful psychological thing as well as a potent source for sensation. As in the scene described below, many people choose to play using knives that have been deliberately dulled to reduce the chance of accidental injury, particularly when the genitals are to be involved. This is a great idea, particularly since the genitals are not nearly sensitive enough in the right ways to tell whether the blade is dull or sharp. In fact, with a blindfolded bottom or with a bottom who is restrained so that he cannot see the area you are tormenting, many implements feel just like knives with hardly any of the risk: thin-bladed icing spreaders are a great option, and believe it or not, the edge of a metal spoon can elicit just as much response as a switchblade if your playmate has been primed to think that that's exactly what it is.

If you do choose to play with a sharp knife, make sure it is a knife you know well and know how to handle. Single-edged blades are much safer than double-edged blades, having only half the cutting surface. (Note: double-edged blades, such as switchblades, are illegal in many places. Check your local laws if you own, or plan to acquire, any such knives.) Single-bladed knives are also much more versatile and easy to use for play, since the back of a single-edged blade is a safe and very effective thing to use for sensation play in any knife play scene.

Something to keep foremost in your mind, should you decide to play with sharp blades, is that a truly sharp blade will cut with little or no pain. Often, you may not even realize you've broken the skin until you see the blood. I once teased the tip of a new knife across the back of my hand, expecting to experience just an enjoyable light tingly scratching sensation. A moment later I was bleeding quite profusely from a three-inch-long (but fortunately very shallow) cut that I hadn't even felt, and was rapidly developing a whole new respect for just how sharp the tip of a knife could be. This is not something you want to find out by accident in a scene, and particularly not on someone else's body or genitals.

Be aware that not everyone can deal with knives used in BDSM play, and even those who don't mind knife play in other scene contexts may not be prepared to handle it in cock and ball play scenarios. The fear of castration that comes along with having a knife near a man's genitals can be pretty extreme, so be careful and compassionate as you play, and don't surprise someone with knife play. Negotiate it, or don't do it.

Much more innocuous, but no less effective, is *Velcro*. Available at your local camping goods or sewing shop, the bristly side, made up of hundreds of small plastic hooks, is very useful for sensation play. It can be lightly rubbed or more firmly scoured against the skin, or trailed lightly over it to produce a variety of sensations. It is very abrasive, however, so keep an eye out for signs that you may have rubbed too hard or traumatized the skin.

In Context

Your partner, a bottom, has been hinting about his love of rope lately, and you know he has a couple of steamy fantasies involving cowboys and the Wild, Wild West – a combination bound to give a person a few interesting ideas. So you discuss it a bit.

How does he feel about having his cock and balls all tied up with rope? Pretty damned good, as it turns out. How about being put in body bondage as well as genital bondage? He just smiles and nods and spreads his arms as if begging you to spread-eagle him. What about a little bit of pain? His grin gets wider, but he reminds you that "a little" means just that, and you smile, remind him of his safeword, and agree. Finally, you ask him whether it'd be okay to use a knife in the scene. He knows you've got an ongoing fascination with knives. He looks a little unsure, but he trusts you, and he knows you know what you're doing. Plus, he's feeling a little adventurous, so he says okay, but he doesn't want any blood play. You don't either, so it works out wonderfully, and in short order the two of you are off to a great start on a fabulous evening's play.

Your partner strips out of his clothes, and then, on your orders, he puts his boots back on. While he is changing, you remove your shirt, slip a pair of Western chaps over your jeans, and put on tall brown cowboy boots. You wrap tie a black bandanna around your neck, and toss a coil of your favorite cock-and-ball bondage rope over your shoulder. You slip a pair of clamp-on spurs onto your heels for the wonderful jingling sound they make, and when you straighten back up, you realize that your partner is kneeling naked before you. An obliging lad, he nuzzles your crotch through the jeans. After he licks your boots for a while, you pick him up (well, figuratively speaking!) and toss him onto your four-poster bed, where four short lengths of rope you keep tied to the posts "just in case!" provide you with the means to quickly and comfortably spread-eagle your willing captive.

Climbing onto the bed, you straddle your partner's torso, alternately massaging and slapping his chest. As his body slowly gets accustomed to the sensations, you increase the intensity a little in short flurries of slaps to his pecs, and then, slowly, you begin to move down his body – but not to his cock and balls. No, first the insides of his thighs get the same kind of treatment you gave his pecs, kneading and slapping, first soft, then more firm.

Once his legs are quivering and reddened from slapping, you gently stroke his cock and balls, just letting him become used to your touch.

Finally you grab his scrotum, right at the base of his cock. Slowly but firmly you pull it away from his body, using first one hand and then the other, gently stretching it, tugging it like your favorite taffy in the world, loosening it up a little and slowly stretching it away from his body. By now he is moaning, his cock is stiff, and he has started to squirm, so it's clearly time for the fun to begin.

Taking the coil of thin, flexible rope from your shoulder, you unwind it so that you have the full eight-foot length to play with. Holding about a foot of rope in your left hand, you position it at the base of his cock. Working nice and slow so that he feels every inch of rope as it wraps around his flesh, you begin to wrap the rope around the base of his cock and balls, just as if it were a cock ring. Wrapping carefully to avoid pulling out pubic hair, you cinch up the first few turns... then begin wrapping the top of your playmate's scrotum in exactly the same way, forming a handsome rope ball stretcher to go with the nice rope cock ring he's just acquired. After about five to six wraps with the rope, you tie off the rope in a half hitch or bow knot, keeping the short end – the slip end of the knot that you can pull to release the knot – in your hand.

What to do with the remainder of the rope, that five or six feet of line that dangles onto the bed? Well, you pull it up toward your partner's mouth, tugging it tight and forcing the rope between his teeth so that his cock and balls are red and engorged with blood, and he, lucky boy, is forced to hold himself by the balls with his teeth. He has ceased struggling, and watches you closely as you circle the bed, wondering what is going to happen next. Reaching into your boot you pull out a large Bowie knife, which you toss casually from hand to hand, feeling the weight and balance. Light reflects off the gleaming blade, making patterns on the ceiling and walls. His eyes are fixed on the knife.

You move closer to the bed, still passing the knife from hand to hand. You grasp the handle of the knife firmly and slowly move the shining blade toward his red, throbbing cock. Carefully, you press the flat side of the blade against his swollen balls. It is cold and makes him want to jerk away, but he is aware of the knife's potential danger and resists his urge to retreat. He also has that rope in his mouth, and even a slight flinch gives him a firm tug at the other end, and it serves as a pretty good reminder!

Now that you have his full attention, you turn the knife around. You grasp one of his curling pubic hairs between your thumb and the back of the blade, keeping the edge away from his body. You watch his eyes as you quickly yank the hair out by the roots, and listen with a wicked grin as he groans. His breath begins to come in quick pants as the pain of the pulled hair fuels the sexual excitement already burning inside him. So you add another log to that fire, yanking another hair free, and watch his body twitch from the sensation. Almost uncontrollably a smile spreads across your face as you look into his eyes and see a combination of excitement, love, and a building rage from the teasing pain.

After plucking out a few more hairs, you hold his balls in your hands. Using the point of the knife, you touch the stretched skin of his scrotum.

The reaction is what you had hoped for. Yelping and panting, he cringes and cries out every time you graze his balls with the tip of the knife. Though you are getting more and more excited yourself, you're careful to remember the limit you agreed upon in negotiations: no blood. From experience you know just how much pressure you can put on the knife's point before it breaks the skin, but you also have a little secret: this knife has been specially prepared for scene play. The edge of the blade has been dulled enough to make an accidental cut almost impossible. But your partner sure doesn't know that, and cold steel, either sharp or dull, feels the same on the genitals.

He's panting hard, now, so you decide to calm him down... the hard way. You lay the knife on his heaving stomach with the point aimed toward his cock. His panting slows, as the fear of jostling the knife and accidentally cutting himself forces him to slow his breathing.

"That's it," you say encouragingly, and you pull out another short piece of rope, about three feet in length. This is for his cock. You start at the glans, or head, and lay a short length of rope along the length of the cock toward his balls. Holding the rope at the base you begin wrapping the shaft with rope. Each turn of the rope encircles both the cock and the short length of rope that runs down the length of the shaft. This bit of rope helps keep the winding secure as you work your way up the length of his shaft. Then, when you reach the end of his cock, you tie the two ends of the rope together in a slipknot. His cock is still stiff as a steel rod, but now it is encased in coils of rope.

You pick up the knife again, but this time you put it back in its scabbard. It is out of the scene for now. Climbing up on the bed, you straddle his torso, but this time your ass is in his face so you can concentrate on the exposed tip of his penis. Here's where you get to bring a little modern technology into the mix – reaching into your pocket and pulling out a short piece of Velcro, the rough, bristly side with the tiny plastic hooks. For the next few minutes you gently rub the head of his cock with the rough surface of the Velcro… lightly and then less lightly, teasing him so that it seems like hours instead of minutes. After just a few strokes, he is panting again, and occasionally letting out uncontrollable yelps of sensation and desire.

"Noisy, ain't'cha?" you laugh, pushing your ass into his face to stifle his racket. As you keep tormenting his cock-head you feel him nuzzle into the denim of your jeans and muffle his own screams. After a while, your own arousal gets the better of you and you decide to segue out of the cock and ball play part into some more traditional and typical gratification… and after all is said and done and all the ropes are untied, you can almost hear the other cowboys snoring in the bunkhouse as your partner snuggles up against your chest and you both drift off for a well-satisfied nap.

Swing Low

Equipment
small doeskin flogger
bamboo skewers
twitch
chain
spring snaps (also called "panic snaps")
weights

Techniques
When using a *flogger* on someone's cock and balls, the important thing to keep in mind is how hard you are hitting. As with the technique for using a rubber or "bungee" flogger discussed in earlier sections, holding the man's cock or balls in your hand and making sure that you

hit your hand in the process is a good way to be aware of how hard you are hitting.

A lightweight and very soft doeskin flogger, particularly one of the small ones sold as "hip whips," "dick whips," or "pussy whips," is highly unlikely to be able to deliver a blow hard enough to do any physical damage. This may not be the case with heavier floggers with sharper or less flexible tails, so be aware of the limitations of whatever implement you choose.

For technique advice on using *bamboo skewers*, please see the technique section of the "Double Your Pleasure" section.

Twitches, sometimes sold as "ball crushers," are used to clamp around the skin of the scrotum between the testicles and the body. In their closed position, they will rest on the testicles, with the weight of the twitch stretching the scrotum somewhat and holding the testicles at the bottom of the scrotum. Because twitches are made of metal and thus will not stretch, they are an excellent fixture from which to hang weights on the scrotum without worrying that the fixture itself might stretch, allowing one or both testicles to slip through the opening, which could be extremely painful and injurious. This is a potential liability with parachutes, and one of the reasons that twitches are a better choice if you want to hang weights from someone's scrotum (or your own).

Weights for cock and ball play are a matter of personal taste – and endurance! Before I say anything else about using weights, let me just say this: cock and ball play, like BDSM generally, is not a competition. Doing more, heavier weights doesn't make you better than the next guy, it just increases the chances that you're going to hurt yourself. The body will tell you what it can take and what it wants, if you let it. Tension, sleep or lack of it, emotional state, and many other factors come into play in the complex interrelationship of mind and body. Sometimes this means that you might not be able to take as much as you did the last time you played, and that's okay. Sometimes it may mean that you can take more than you ever dreamed possible. If you can be in the moment with your body as you play, you will know what's right for you.

The technique of hanging weights from someone's genitals is both simple and requires practice and attention. There are two basic principles.

The first is start light and work your way up. It is always possible to add more weight if it is desired. It is very difficult to back off successfully if you have begun with something that has already pushed over a limit or caused "bad pain." The mood will be broken, and the scene will basically be over before it has much of a chance to begin. On the other hand, if you have an assortment of weights of different sizes, and begin with small ones and work your way up (in the "In Context" section, you'll notice that the top first lets the bottom get used to the weight of the twitch alone, then the twitch plus the chain alone, before adding any other weights), you can not only be much more assured of not unintentionally going past a boundary point, but the scene lasts that much longer, too.

The second principle is what my high school gym teacher called "not abusing the weights." Never let them drop suddenly, and never let them fall with their full weight against one another (no matter how much you like that loud clanking sound!). This is to avoid tearing the tissues of the genitals to which those weights are attached. Human tissues such as skin are amazingly resilient if you stretch them slowly. If you don't, on the other hand, you can damage or tear them remarkably easily, possibly causing permanent damage. This is something to be careful of not only when attaching weights, but when moving them around after you've attached them. Any time you swing a weight, you're exerting torque on the genitals, a force which may be commensurate to many times the actual poundage of the weights themselves, so be aware.

For attaching weights to the genitals, you need something to attach them to, and something to attach or hang them with. Weights can be put on a number of different kinds of "fixtures," including twitches, ball stretchers, cock and ball harnesses, parachutes, and cock rings. Weights can also be attached to clips or clamps, but beware: too much weight can pull a clip or clamp off, which may or may not be desirable.

Depending on the size of the weight, different means for hanging weights are appropriate. For very small weights, a small wire S-hook works well (unbend a heavy-duty paperclip in the middle and you have one in your hand!). For medium-sized weights, a double-ended panic snap is a good option, or a heavier-duty metal S-hook works well too. For heavier weights or dumbbell plates with a hole through their middles, attaching a chain to the "fixture" with a panic snap, then threading the chain through the weights and securing the loose end of the chain to the portion above the weights with a second panic snap is a great option.

When you remove weights, make sure to lift up the weight in one hand, taking the the weight off of the genitals, before you remove the weight from its attachment point. The manipulations you have to make on the attachment point may otherwise cause the weight to exert unwelcome torque, potentially causing pain as well as making actually more difficult to remove the weight. This is particularly true in any instance where you need to remove weights quickly. It may seem quicker to do it without lifting the weight first, but in this case, haste makes waste.

In Context

You and your submissive partner – your "boy," as he's called in the scene, though he's very much a man – are going to a dungeon party. Being a bit of an exhibitionist, he would like you to do a cock and ball play scene with him there. Being a bit of an exhibitionist yourself you agree, and pack a small (and heavy!) toy bag for the occasion. You will do a variation on a scene that you and your boy have done several times before in private, knowing that the results will be both predictable and wonderful.

Arriving at the party with the early guests, you give your leather jacket to your boy and tell him to go get dressed in the outfit you gave him to wear. While you chat with friends, he hangs up your jacket and retires to the back room to change. He returns in a few minutes in his combat boots and a leather harness, an arrangement of straps and chrome rings that crisscrosses his chest, outlining his pecs and emphasizing his broad shoulders. A thick strap descends to his waist from the ring at the center of his chest, joining a ring at the waist from which several straps branch out to a leather waistband, and a single strap leads down to a cock ring. From the rear, two straps pass around his butt and through the legs like a jock strap. These attach to the bottom of the cock ring, pulling it taut against his body and lifting his cock and balls slightly.

Festively attired, your boy sits attentively at your feet while you finish a conversation with a close friend who just happens to be a well-known dominatrix. You are aware of your partner's eagerness, so you draw out the conversation a bit just to see him fidget. Finally, though, you decide that it is time. You toss your boy the toy bag and start toward the playroom.

The playroom is busy, but the Saint Andrew's Cross, a large X made of framing timbers, is vacant. From another corner you can hear the rhythmic slapping of a riding crop against skin as you point to the big wooden cross. Your boy knows what to do, and mounts the cross, lying with his back against the timbers and raising his hands above his head, laying them out along the uprights. You shackle his hands using the padded cuffs attached to the cross, the heavy metal buckles jingling appealingly as you secure them. Nudging his feet apart, you strap the leg shackles on his ankles and snap them to the short chains at the base of the cross. He is now spread-eagled, very vulnerable, well-restrained, and delightfully aroused at the thought of what is to come.

A few people gather at a respectful distance to watch. They have heard about your play, and one of the wonderful things about parties like this is that they offer chances for folks in the scene to see other players work. You like the thought of them watching you as you put your boy through his paces, and the little purr of exhibitionist pleasure makes you grin. Your boy likes it too, so you put a leather blindfold on him – all the better to let him wonder how many pairs of eyes are on him, plus it makes well-timed surprises that much easier. Besides, he's told you that he enjoys the experience of the minor disorientation he gets from being blindfolded, as well as the way it cuts out visual distractions. For yourself, you will have to use all your concentration to focus on your boy and the scene without being distracted by the scenes around you. You can still enjoy the energy of the room, but as long as the scene lasts, the sole item of your attention is your boy.

"Remember what I say to you," you say as you adjust his blindfold. "If you feel we are going too fast, you will tell me. You will say, 'Please Sir, may I catch my breath, Sir?'"

He nods. This is his "caution word." It doesn't mean he wants to stop, just that he needs to slow down a little.

"And if we are doing something that might injure you, or things get too intense and you want to stop, you will say, 'Please Sir, may we stop for now, Sir?' There is no shame in doing this. I would be unhappy if you weren't honest, do you understand?"

He smiles and nods. He knows you are reinforcing the bonds of trust you have built together. Having a safeword or phrase gives him the option of ending any scene for any reason. With a cock and ball play scene, safewords are particularly important, because where such delicate body parts are involved, almost any play means there's at least some potential for damage, and the more intense the play, the more significant the risk.

Before you step away from him you kiss him hard on the mouth, an intimate gesture that seals your commitment as his top, and grab his beefy pecs for a rough squeeze. You love to hear the intake of breath as he gives himself over to your sensations. Then you turn away to open the toy bag and lay out your tools for the evening.

First on the menu is a small doeskin flogger. This will be used for a warm up, since its tails are soft and very pliable, and despite the startling, stimulating loud pop they can make, they can cause no real damage even when swung at full force. For the next course, you lay out a small bundle of bamboo cooking skewers. These, when slapped against the skin, can deliver a deep sting to the penis, balls or just about any other part of the anatomy. They are the miniature equivalent of a cane, and when used with force can raise welts, but they also work nicely as sensation playthings for poking, stroking and tickling.

On to the entrée! You remove a twitch from the bag, a heavy metal vise-like device your boy loves, and along with it comes a heavy chain, several chrome spring snaps, and then a few different sizes of deep sea fishing weights. And for dessert, the heavy artillery: four two and one-half pound plates from a dumbbells set. A few of the onlookers gasp when they see these. You chuckle to yourself, remembering the first time you saw weights as heavy as these used in a cock and ball scene. You almost fainted then, but now you love the effect they have on your boy, and, more importantly, so does he.

You reach out for your boy's semi-rigid cock and run your fingers along the silky shaft. His breathing is loud and deep, and you can tell that he is using all his restraint to keep from getting rock hard right away. After you toy with him a bit, you hold his cock in your open left palm, enjoying the feel and the weight of it in your hand. Using the doeskin flogger, you start with a few light strokes. The tails hit both his cock and your hand, this way you can judge the severity of the blows and gauge how fast you will accelerate the intensity.

Your boy is smiling as you do this. The doeskin always tickles at first. Then there's a harder slap, and his smile vanishes as he has to catch his breath. This little flogger can't do any damage, but it sure can sting! After a few more slaps, you lift his cock up and start to work on the balls, first with lighter strokes, but then increasing the intensity as he gets used to the sensation. With each slap you watch his body jerk as he fights his natural instinct to pull away from you. He enjoys the sharp sting of the whip on his balls, though, and in a few minutes, you have him panting as he is tugged back and forth between pain and pleasure. Each stroke of the flogger hurts, yes, but it also releases a wave of endorphins that make him shiver.

Once you've got your boy well warmed up, you set the doeskin flogger down and press your cheek to his, listening to his short rapid breaths. You whisper encouragement into his ear, along with a reassurance that you will let him settle down a little before continuing.

Once his breathing has resumed its normal rhythm, you pick up the bamboo skewers. One in each hand, you press the points lightly against the skin of his neck. Then, with a slow sweeping motion, you trace the contours of his body all the way to his feet. It sends shivers through him and you smile, pleased by his responsiveness.

Again lifting his cock in your hand, you feel it start to swell with blood. Using two skewers in one hand, you begin lightly tapping the head of his cock with the shafts of the slim bamboo rods. This light action is not painful at first, but as you continue the action for what seems like hours to him, the repeated light strokes become cumulative in their action. They don't sting so much as they annoy. That is the game now, to annoy him to the brink of anger, and then back off. It works wonders. Finally he can contain himself no longer and he starts growling and roaring like an animal. Such a simple action, yet such a primal, visceral result!

As you did before, you caress him and give him time to recover. He is sweating profusely, and you lick some of the salty drops from his chest before turning your attention to his balls. The chill in the room has caused his nuts to tighten and withdraw toward the warmth of his body. Gently easing them away from his body, you slowly pull them with your fingers in a firm, fist-like grip, stretching the skin of the scrotum gently, persistently loosening him up for the main event.

Taking a break from your ministrations, you reach behind you and pick up the twitch, a device sometimes referred to as a ball crusher, and drop it on the floor in front of him. He can't see it, of course, but the heavy metal clank gets his attention. It also gets the attention of several people in the room who have been watching your play. Cock and ball play both fascinates and frightens some people, and the thought of a cold metal instrument like the twitch being used on something as delicate and personal as someone's balls is quite enough to give some people a bad case of the chills. But the onlookers aren't the only ones: your boy is shivering too, but without a trace of worry, only eager anticipation and a hint of a smile.

You start by opening the clamp to its full width and dropping his balls in between its jaws. Making sure you have gathered all the loose skin of his scrotum in your fist, you begin to tighten the device, slowly tightening it around the expanse of loose skin between the body and the testicles. The twitch you use is made of heavy aluminum, and will only tighten down so far – not far enough to do any harm to his scrotum, but tight enough that his testicles can't slip through, which makes it very suitable as a fixture for hanging weights. With a parachute or other device there might be a chance of one or both testicles slipping through the parachute opening when weight was put on the parachute itself, and that would be a scene-stopping event for sure, as well as a painful one. But that can't happen with a twitch. Metal isn't flexible, and it definitely won't stretch.

As you tighten the twitch, you continue to hold the skin of his scrotum gathered, preventing it from getting caught in the sliding portion of the clamp. You want his nuts intact when you are through so you can play again. Your boy groans slightly as the twitch reaches its fully closed position and you let the weight of the device hang fully on his balls. You like the way the shiny metal looks framing his nuts, and you start it swinging gently to catch the light. As you swing it back and forth, he again groans in pleasure.

Now the real test of his mettle — or was that metal? — begins. You take a short piece of chain and thread it through the handle of the twitch. As you slowly let the weight of the chain add to the weight of the twitch itself, you watch his face to see if it is having its desired effect. He is still smiling and groaning every so often, so you know that it is.

You play a while with the chain, letting it clink back and forth, occasionally brushing his inner thighs with it as you swing it in a slow circle. You love to watch the reaction of his skin to the cold metal chain. The goose bumps are magical, and you enjoy watching his body's involuntary changes as you play with him.

But now it's time for the heavy stuff, literally as well as figuratively. Since your boy is experienced with this game, and since you've done this with him many times and know he loves heavy weights, you start with a two and a half pound dumbbell plate. Threading the chain through the plate and locking the loop of chain to itself with a spring snap, you slowly lower the dumbbell plate until the full weight is pulling on your partner's balls. Behind you hear a man gasp. Turning, you see a man in a harness and collar cowering at the feet of a tall black dominatrix. He looks up at her, and when she looks down and smiles, he crawls behind her legs in fear. This is not for the meek.

You drop a second steel plate on the floor. The thud makes your boy shiver again. With quick, practiced movements you open the spring clamp and thread the second plate on the chain. You slowly lower the steel disk, and once its full weight is dangling from your boy's nuts, you nudge it a bit so that it clanks against the other plate. The sounds coming from your boy's mouth change as you add weight to his balls. He still groans, but deeper, more primal as you progress, the anguish still audible, but almost an outright moan of pleasure.

You only have one more dumbbell plate with you, and you lift the two dangling plates to relieve the strain while you add the third. This one he will definitely feel. Once the weight is threaded on the chain you hold the other two plates and let the third slide down the chain slowly, rasping against the links until it clangs loudly against the ones in your hand. Both you and your boy love the sound of metal against metal, and the sound almost makes you shiver.

As you lower the weights and the full strain is put on his scrotum you hear it start: that low deep moan that turns into a guttural growl, and finally a deep raspy maniacal laughter. Your boy has transcended his human self and become something completely different. He laughs deeply in that voice that seems to billow up from his soul, and you stand there feeling awed by the transformation taking place right in front of you. It is magical!

And you too are transformed. You take no notice of anyone around you. It is just you and your boy. You are drawing his energy now, and your laughter joins his as he swings the weights back and forth from his balls. In a few minutes, he is slowing down and you know it is time to release him. You begin removing the weights, letting each drop loudly on the floor as you take it off the chain. The twitch comes off last, and after it is off, you massage his aching balls gently and lovingly in your hand. His cock has been erect and dripping throughout the scene, and you know he has enjoyed your work.

You can feel his legs vibrating slightly as you undo the cuffs around his ankles, and he collapses into your arms as you uncuff his wrists. You lower him to the floor, cradling him in your arms as you slowly remove the blindfold and look into his teary eyes. He is beginning to return to his body, and you see how deeply you have touched his soul. Scenes like these make you both feel connected beyond any other kind of lovemaking you have known. Through these physical acts, you have communed with the innermost parts of his spirit. Who could ask for more than that?

Spilling the Beans

Equipment

Violet Wand

Technique

The *Violet Wand* is an electrostimulation device designed and originally sold as a quack medicine implement to be used to cure acne, baldness, neuralgia, and the like. It doesn't do any of those things, but what it does do is transform common household current into a high frequency but very low amperage current that can be used to stimulate the skin in various pleasurable and painfully pleasurable ways. Wand-shaped (of course!), the base can be outfitted with a number of different attachments which distribute the current. Some are ball or mushroom-shaped, shaped like rakes, or can be in various other configurations that give varying numbers of points and types of surfaces through which the current may contact the skin. You can experiment with the various attachments available with your Violet Wand to find out which ones you like best. The Violet Wand does not need to be pressed against the skin, however. It will handily produce nice visible sparks that will leap from the Wand to the person you're using it on (turn out the lights for a nice show!).

The high-frequency nature of the current produced by Violet Wands means that the electricity tends to stay in or just under the skin, and is unlikely to go through or do any harm to internal organs. Still, Violet Wands should not be used on the eyes or in any orifice. Using the Violet Wand for prolonged periods, particularly on one area of skin, can result in burns, so move it around and don't zap the same place too often. Also, be careful of using Violet Wands near piercings or metal, such as the metal fittings in a cock harness, for instance. Conductive metals can intensify a shock in an undesirable way, and the same conductive factor can also lead to burns.

One counterintuitive aspect of the Violet Wand is what's called the "distance factor." Holding a Wand an inch or three away from the skin can actually produce a stronger shock than if you were to hold it with the conductive attachment pressed directly against the skin. Why is this? Simply, the farther the electrical charge has to travel, and the more air it must travel through in order to find a ground (the person you are using it on is that ground), the more energy must build up within the Wand before a spark can jump the gap. Also, the larger the conductive attachment you use, the weaker the shock will generally feel: the air inside an attachment acts as a resistor, for one thing, and the broader the surface area of the attachment that comes into contact with the skin the more diffuse the sensation will feel.

In Context

I can't remember the movie, but the scene still is vivid in my mind: a room with stone walls, water dripping from overhead and trickling down the walls. Blue light reflected on the wet stones and bounced around the room, shimmering like the beams of moonlight reflected off the surface of a lake. Meat hooks and chains dangled from the ceiling.

It was certainly not a pretty place, even though the delicate blue reflections gave it a mystical air. Then a man was brought in and stripped of his clothes. What followed involved torture with electrical wires by some very evil characters, a scene that was nonconsensual, and scary as hell, but I couldn't take my eyes off of it – it was riveting even though on some level I knew it was just a movie, not real.

Years later, in a warehouse, electrical "torture" equipment at the ready, I felt the same suspension of disbelief, the same tingle of fear and excitement. This time wasn't any more "real" than that movie had been – it was a scene, and a consensual one, arranged in advance by a friend of mine as an elaborate Christmas gift for his lover – but every instant of the "abduction" and "interrogation" and even the "torture" was riveting, edge-of-your seat fun.

My friend and his lover, Jack, were planning to come into town for Christmas weekend, and together with some mutual friends who were all well-known and could be trusted to play safely and sanely in a highly-charged scene, my friends and I put together a really elaborate piece of cock and ball play theater. Who could resist a Christmas eve consisting of an elaborate set-up, a gorgeous man, and cock and ball play? Not me!

The evening's entertainment was set up as an abduction. Now, this in itself is a very tricky thing to carry out – it's difficult to balance not giving away the surprise without sending the "abductee" into a potentially dangerous panic. And of course, there is always a chance that some suspicious bystander might alert the authorities to what they'd likely see as a highly dangerous and illegal act.

I suppose this is the right time to warn the reader: this is not something I intend for you to try at home! We planned this scene for weeks, and had we not been absolutely sure, based on Jack's own words in many fantasy-sharing emails, that Jack would really get off on the night's festivities, we would have never attempted it at all. Kidnapping is not only a crime, but something which could do serious physical and/or psychological damage. But Jack had been writing stories of erotic abductions and sending them to his lover via email for weeks, and e-mail was their private method of scene negotiation. Jack would write a story for his lover, and if his lover liked the premise, he would help make Jack's fantasies come true. A very considerate lover, I must say.

It just so happened that Jack had a particular fantasy about finding a suitcase full of money. Not just any money, but money belonging to a mob boss. In his fantasy, he had kept the suitcase, figuring that so much cash was ill gotten booty, only to be found out and kidnapped by the mob boss, who tortures him until he talks. In Jack's story, the boss turned out to be gay, and after Jack spilled the beans, the mob boss decided to keep Jack as his personal sex slave. Hot material for a fantasy… and a great basic script for the group of us who were going to carry it out for his Christmas treat!

The night of the big event, Jack's lover brought him to the local leather bar, where he was in collar and following a highly formal protocal of ritualized submission. His lover had discussed giving him to another Top for the evening as a Christmas gift, and Jack was noticeably excited about the possibility. I had arrived at the bar earlier and met up with two friends I'd enlisted to play my "toadies" for the evening and assist in the kidnapping and interrogation. Walter, a jovial good-natured bottom, would play the part of "Mousey." All Mousey did was chuckle under his breath and breathe very noisily. We imagined him as a combination of Freddie Krueger in *Nightmare On Elm Street* and Lenny in *Of Mice And Men*, a scary combination of sadism and innocence. The other friend was "Geno," an efficient thug ready to do the mob boss's dirty work.

Around 10:00 pm, just before the bar started getting busy, Jack's lover blindfolded him and clipped a leash to his collar. He then walked

Jack out into the cold night air wearing nothing but the harness and jock he had changed into in the bar. Once outside, we closed in. Jack's lover handed me the leash and said in a loud voice, "He's yours for the evening, guys, call my cell phone when you're done."

As Geno and Mousey moved in to flank Jack, his lover whispered in his ear, "Merry Christmas, boy."

I can only imagine what it must've seemed like from Jack's perspective. Hustled into the back seat of a large car, trapped between two large men, with no real idea of where he was going, he had no idea that in the real world, his lover was in the front seat with me as the car pulled out of the parking lot. As I drove, my friends and I kept up a spicy dialogue that had something to do with wanting to get this over with, and being disgusted by yet again having to our boss's dirty work. Jack was beginning to wonder what was going on. This didn't sound like a night with a hot leather Daddy. Maybe our voices weren't the familiar ones he thought they were.

By the time we got to our destination, Jack was shivering noticeably, but whether it was fear, anticipation, or a combination, I can't say. My friend Jim, a wholesaler in the floral industry, had loaned us the use of his warehouse for the evening, and we made a lot of noise in the deserted industrial area as we unrolled the metal door on the loading dock and pushed Jack inside. The door rolled down with a crash, and then there was eerie silence. Jim was there to help, and he and Walter moved Jack over to a chain link wall that divided part of the warehouse. We purposefully let Jack's blindfold slip a little so he could see some of the surroundings, but all the while, Jack's lover made sure to be behind Jack, so he himself couldn't be seen. We could all appreciate the delighted grin on Jack's lover's face. We felt the same way, but couldn't show it. It was like playing make-believe as kids, but with a grownup twist, and we were all having loads of fun.

The room was lit by a single light bulb hanging overhead. We had been by earlier to set the stage, and had removed bulbs from the other warehouse lights for effect.

We spread-eagled Jack against the chain link divider, and put his blindfold back in its place, but not until we were sure he'd gotten a chance to notice the row of car batteries we'd lined up, electrical cables linking them together. These were strictly for show, mind you, but they looked superbly ominous and gave him the hint that something electrical was going to be involved.

In my role as interrogator, I asked him a few questions, most of which were designed to lead him to recall his "captured by a mobster" fantasy. I told him that we knew he had the money, and if he would just tell us where it was, we'd let him go. This was his safeword – if he had not played along we would've known he wasn't clueing into the nature of the game, and we would have let him go instantly. But he seemed to have a pretty good idea of what was going on, and as he answered with a sassy, impertinent "I don't have any money, and if I did, I wouldn't tell you jerks," it became obvious that he knew he was in no danger. No, Jack was enjoying himself, and there was a rapidly-growing lump in his jockstrap providing further evidence.

I slapped him across the face, only hard enough to make a noise, not with enough force to do any damage or do much more than sting for an instant. "Cut that jock off this bastard!" I barked.

Jim took a pair of bandage scissors and quickly cut through the worn fabric of Jack's jock. His cock sprang out like a rocket. If there was any doubt that he didn't know this was a scene it was abundantly clear now. "Well, looks like this guy likes being tied up," I growled. "Geno, give me those wires. Let's see how much he likes *juice*."

Jim handed me a Violet Wand we had hidden behind the batteries. For tonight's fun, the wand had a metal rod attached. Unlike the glass tubes most people use with these harmless toys, the solid metal rod can deliver a hefty but definitely not dangerous zap. The intensity of the shock can be controlled by the rheostat on the base of the unit, making it easy to change as circumstances dictate.

"OK, asshole, now I'm gonna put this wire right up close to your dick, and when it gets close enough, your cock is gonna give us a little fireworks show. That is, unless you tell me where the money is."

"Fuck you!" Jack said with a sneer.

I pushed the button on the wand and touched it to his balls. Zap! A spark jumped from the wand to the skin of his scrotum. Jack reacted with a scream, just as we expected… and then followed up with a string of expletives that gave a clear signal he was getting into this and enjoying the role of the rebellious captive to the hilt. "I told you I'm not gonna tell you where it is," Jack repeated as he squirmed in his bonds.

Zap! Again the wand shot sparks, but this time near the base of his cock. Jack screamed again, and almost climbed the chain link wall backwards. This sequence continued for almost thirty minutes, first a short zap, each time to a different part of his genitalia, then Jack calling me every name in the book but steadfastly refusing to reveal the location of the "money." Throughout the scene his cock stayed rigid, no mean feat, considering that the normal reaction of the genitals to fear and pain is to retreat as far into the body as possible. Clearly, we were doing something right.

Finally, he was getting exhausted, and we thought it was time to give him a break. "Okay, tough guy. If I can't get it out of you with pain, then I guess I'll have to try something else. Geno, Mousey, cut him down!"

Jim and Walter cut the ropes that loosely held Jack against the chain-link fencing. It didn't take long for him to slump to his knees. He was sweating up a storm, but was still vibrating with excitement and arousal when I reached down and took his head in my hands. I cradled it there gently for a few moments, and the turned it upwards, facing directly into my crotch. "All righty, then, you think you're such a stud that even the juice won't get anything out of you, well, let's see just how well you can suck cock, prettyboy."

Jack's body went rigid, and for a moment he resisted. During those few seconds, his lover stepped into my place, his cock already out of his pants and very erect. He moved forward, pushing his dick into Jack's mouth. Jack was hesitant at first, but relented and began going all the way down on his lover's cock. I stepped back and let him continue fantasizing that he was being forced to give head to some strange mobster.

Jim, Walter and I watched the scene in awe. Jack was having a field day, and so was his lover. Before his lover came, he pulled his cock out of Jack's mouth and shot his load down Jack's chest. Jack was stroking his own cock throughout it all, and he exploded shortly afterward.

As Jack was catching his breath, his lover removed the blindfold from his eyes. Jack blinked and looked up, his face showing both surprise and relief. "Merry Christmas, boy," his lover said through a thousand-watt smile. "Geno" and "Mousey" and Jim and I joined them, pulling out Christmas cookies and hot cocoa and pulling up seats together on the floor, reminiscing about the hot scene we'd just played, a wonderfully seasonal ending to a fantastic night.

Getting the Point
Equipment & Technique

After some deliberation, I decided to include this scene because of the growing popularity of temporary piercing, also known as "play piercing." This is not intended as a step-by-step guide to this kind of play, but rather a glimpse at how temporary piercing can be incorporated into cock and ball play to create an extraordinary scene. Having said this, I want to make it clear that I recommend that you DO NOT try this yourself… at least until you have gotten some serious and in-depth personal instruction from someone experienced in piercing and the precautions and procedures necessary to minimize risks. This is why there is not a detailed equipment list or commentary for this section, as there has been for previous ones. I do not intend for you to use this scenario as a "recipe," but merely as a source for information and, perchance, as something to urge you to go and learn more.

For more detailed information about temporary piercings I would refer the reader to Trevor Jacques' *On the Safe Edge*. This book is currently out of print (as of the time of this writing), but you can surely find someone in your local BDSM community who will lend you a copy. While you're at it you can surely ask around for someone to help you learn to do play piercing safely!

Any scene involving invasive activities such as piercing requires a good knowledge of the activity itself and the techniques you need to do it, but the possible repercussions of the activity as well. Any time you break the skin, you open up a tiny door to the interior of the body. This door is all it takes for an infection to invade. The human body is covered with lots of microorganisms and bacteria that are harmless to us as long as they are outside our bodies, but given a direct access to the body's interior and the bloodstream, they can be not only pesky, but dangerous.

To minimize the risk of unwanted infection in a play piercing scene, a number of precautions can and should be taken. First and foremost, use only sterile, single-use disposable needles. These can be obtained from surgical supply houses or veterinary supply companies. Needles come in many different sizes, from very thin short needles for injecting insulin (which are not suitable for play piercing, because they are fragile and may break or bend) to extremely large needles used in surgical procedures. I prefer needles between 22 and 25 gauge for cock and ball play piercing scenes. These are long enough and stiff enough not to bend when you least expect it, and still thin enough to not to cause too much pain or damage the skin beyond a tiny hole.

The tips of hypodermic needles are cut at an angle, creating a very efficient device for piercing the skin. In temporary piercing, the object is to create a hole that will heal almost immediately, unlike the kind of piercing done when a piece of jewelry is going to be left behind. Hypodermic needles are helpful for this, since they do not punch a hole in the skin but rather push it out of the way.

Second, you will need a "sharps container," a hard plastic container designed to resist the points of needles and other sharp items. These can be purchased at drug stores in many places, but an alternative is to use a hard molded plastic bottle, such as the heavyweight opaque bottles in which detergents, bleach, or some kinds of orange juice are sold. A standard two-liter soda bottle is not adequate to the task, you need something sturdier. When a sharps container is full, it is sealed and disposed of. I recommend using packing tape or duct tape to tape the lid onto the container, to prevent someone removing it thoughtlessly or accidentally. Ask your drug store what specific regulations are in effect in your area about the disposal of infectious waste. You don't want any trash handlers getting an accidental needle stick, and possibly an infection, from your carelessness!

Butterfly boards can be made in a few ways. What they all have in common is that they are single-use items. You make one, you use one, you throw it away. Butterfly boards can be one-piece, with a hole in the middle to bring the cock and balls up through, or two-piece, somewhat like a stocks, with the two halves being secured around the cock and balls. In either case, you will want to make your butterfly board out of two thicknesses of foamcore board, or else out of one thickness of plywood topped with one thickness of foamcore board. Needles will go into the top layer of the butterfly board only.

Cleanliness is very important. Prior to beginning the piercing scene, I have my bottom clean the skin of his genitals well with an antibacterial soap and dry the area with a clean towel. I position the bottom on his back, on a comfortable surface (here is where owning an old medical table comes in handy!). The cock and balls are then positioned through the butterfly board (if need be, the halves of the board are tied together, as well as being secured to the bottom's body if need be to help keep it in position). To avoid the body's natural defense mechanism of retracting the testicles during threat or fear reactions, I sometimes put my bottom in a cockring prior to the scene.

I then use Betadine on a sterile piece of gauze or a sterile cotton swab to clean the skin surface of the penis and scrotum. I apply the cleanser using a circular motion, working from the center outward. I then allow this to air dry while I am preparing the needles for the scene. The needles will need to be removed from the paper envelopes they come in and set out on a clean secure surface. I like to use a clean paper towel on a medical instrument tray, but a TV tray or other portable stand will work as well. Just keep everything close and clean. This stand should also have the sharps container on it for easy disposal of the needles.

Sterile surgical gloves are to be preferred for play piercing, but clean fresh surgical gloves straight from the box are acceptable. Change gloves frequently. I suggest changing them after cleaning your bottom's genitals with Betadine, then again after you insert the needles, so that you end up using at least 3 pairs of gloves over the course of the scene. Once you have gloves on, be sure not to touch anything that has not been disinfected. This means not touching your own skin, hair, clothes, or face, your bottom's skin (except for the disinfected skin of his cock and balls), hair, or clothes, and certainly not touching any objects aside from those that have been sterilized for use in the scene. This means that if you need to scratch your nose, you change your gloves. Want a drink of water? Change your gloves before you go back to business. This will help you avoid transmitting foreign microorganisms to your equipment or your bottom's skin.

One of the hazards for the top in a play piercing scene is an accidental needle stick. Use care to avoid pricking yourself with the needles both before and especially after the scene. Because of this possibility, I strongly suggest not trying to put the needles back into the plastic sheaths before discarding them. That is what the sharps container is for! Recapping needles is no longer done in surgery or medical procedures because of this hazard. Simply drop a used needle directly into the sharps container.

When piercing the scrotum or the penis, care must be taken to avoid the larger blood vessels or any irregularities on or in the skin of the penis or scrotum. You will usually be able to tell where larger blood vessels are by looking. Play piercing scenes require adequate bright light. Remember, there's a reason that operating rooms are amazingly well-lit!

During a butterfly scene, needles are inserted through the skin and into the foamcore board below in one smooth motion. Angle the needles slightly away from the scrotum as you insert them. This will help keep the skin slightly taut, and will also help avoid the possibility of skin tension pulling needles out of the foamcore board. Work symmetrically, first placing a needle on one side, then on the other. This helps balance pressure, sensation, and tension on the skin of the scrotum.

Needles are used to penetrate the skin ONLY. Never insert a needle into the spongy tissue of the penis, into or through the urethra, or into the testicle, epididimis, or any other body within the scrotum. The spacing of needles will be dependent upon how many needles you have chosen to use for your scene. More needles will require that they be placed closer together. Fewer needles will require that they be spaced farther apart.

I generally do not use more than a dozen or so needles on someone for whom play piercing is a new activity. The sensations are very intense, and when you add the fear factor, the potential for a bottom to become overstimulated can be significant. By working slowly and calmly, I minimize the bottom's fears and allow him to adjust to the sensation with each insertion of a needle. The body's endorphin pump works overtime during scenes like these, so I like to get feedback from my play partner constantly. Keeping the line of communication open helps me to calm them and gives me important information on how they are responding to the scene.

Each needle should be removed with one continuous smooth movement. They go immediately into the sharps container. After all the needles are removed I once more clean the areas that have been pierced with Betadine, or if I am in a particularly sinister mood, a combination of Betadine and rubbing alcohol. The sting from the alcohol is a little extra treat!

Most of the needle sites will not bleed. If they do, I swab them with an extra sterile alcohol swab after the bleeding has stopped. Usually there won't be more than a drop or two, and the blood coming out actually helps clean out any extraneous material that might have gotten in. I have never encountered any profuse bleeding during a play piercing scene, but I would have no qualms about seeking medical attention should that occur.

I tell the bottom to check the area when he gets home, and again the next morning, just to make sure there is no additional bleeding. I also tell them to clean the area with an antibacterial soap the following morning just to be on the safe side.

It is not uncommon for a bottom to feel slightly dizzy or high after a play piercing scene, so don't rush the aftercare. I try to give bottoms plenty of time to come down and adjust to reality again. This can take a few minutes or several hours, depending on how they respond to their own endorphins and to the scene. I once ended up driving one friend home after doing a piercing scene with him at a play party. Two hours later, he was still feeling very "endorphin high" and I wasn't sure that he was really okay to drive. As the top, I felt a whole lot better knowing that he had been safely tucked in for the night than I would've had he gone out onto the road when he wasn't completely in possession of his full faculties. Checking with him the following morning, I learned he was fine and grateful for the extra measure of aftercare.

In Context

A friend of yours who has always admired your talent in the field of cock and ball play has finally come around to asking you if you would treat him to an example of your handiwork – something very special that he's always wanted to try. You are going to do your favorite kind of edge play scene, a butterfly. This involves using hypodermic needles to pin down the skin of the scrotum, stretching it out into a shape resembling a butterfly. He's a bit nervous, and you understand his fear. The first time you were butterflied, you were afraid, too. In this case, you know fear will make the scene more intense and the experience more memorable for him, but you also know that you've done these scenes many times, have a lot of experience, know what to look out for, and thus, he really has nothing to fear.

Once he is comfortably naked, you have him lie on your medical examining table. It's a great tool for BDSM scenes and a real conversation piece that you've enjoyed ever since you found it at an auction. When it isn't in use, you cover it with a flat plank top and a tablecloth. To those who aren't in the know, it looks like a buffet table. Tonight, however, it puts your friend and playmate at the perfect height for you to work on him.

You have supplies in the drawers below the table. One drawer contains several boxes of disposable hypodermic needles, which you order them from a veterinary supply company. For this scene you need about thirty needles, so you count them out, remove the wrapping but not the plastic sheaths that cover the needles, and place them on a nearby table that you've covered with a sterile, disposable paper towel from your local surgical supply house. In the same drawer are sterile surgical gloves and a few other goodies from the surgical supply, including a bottle of Betadine, some cotton swabs, and some more of those disposable prepackaged sterile towels.

The only other piece of equipment you need is something you make yourself. It is the pin-board or butterfly board: a twelve-inch square of two layers of three-sixteenths-inch (3/16 of an inch) foam-core board, in which you have cut a small central circular hole just big enough for a cock and balls to squeeze through comfortably. You take the pin-board and put it down over your friend's cock, then carefully work his equipment up through the board so that both balls and cock protrude on the topside.

You spray the board with a mist of alcohol as a precaution against surface bacteria. Alcohol will not kill everything, but these boards are fresh and clean and are discarded at the end of the scene, never reused. This way, the chances of infection are slim.

Only now, after putting on a pair of surgical gloves, you are ready to start preparing your partner for the procedure. You use a cotton swab to give his scrotum a good wipedown with Betadine. This surgical pre-wash is used in many operation rooms to prepare the skin before surgery. It minimizes the number of bacteria on the surface of the skin and helps prevent infection. The only downside is the yellowish stain it leaves the skin, but this washes off later.

After this preparation and before you begin the scene itself, you change into a fresh pair of gloves. You lay your forearm reassuringly across your friend's chest, looking into his eyes and assuring him that this will be an experience he will remember, and that you are confident he will come through it just fine. You also warn him that he should remain still, so as not to incur any accidental injuries during the procedure.

Taking the first needle, you hold the sheath in your teeth, and pull the needle out quickly with you hand. Spitting the sheath on the floor, you use your left hand to pull a bit of skin from the scrotum away from his cock, laying it flat against the board. Holding it down between your thumb and forefinger, you push the needle through his skin, pinning it down against the board in one smooth action, being careful not to penetrate both layers of the board. Though you know it doesn't hurt as much as it would seem, your friend is shivering and a little frayed. You speak to him confidently and again lay your forearm across his chest to comfort him. Using your forearm to touch him lets you avoid the possibility of getting germs from his skin on your gloves, possibly causing problems down the road.

When he has calmed down, you repeat the procedure with the area of skin a half-inch or so down the scrotum from the first puncture. He once again starts shivering, but he has a nervous smile on his face. You continue working, stretching and pinning the skin of his balls, shifting from one side to the other of his scrotum, to keep the scene symmetrical. The scene takes on a musical rhythm: lifting the needle, removing the sheath, stretching the skin, inserting the needle. The movements are like a dance, well rehearsed and deliberate. Your pauses to comfort your friend fall into the rhythm too. The whole scene is a careful slow-motion ballet.

With each pin, his endorphins are pumping faster and he is getting higher and higher, until he is almost giddy. You pause every so often to let him absorb the feelings and process the pain. Soon his balls are spread like a giant butterfly pinned down in a collector's display case. You ask if he would like to see, and he nods yes. You use your forearm to assist him is raising his head so he can see the stretched out skin of his balls outlined by twenty needles.

He is astounded, and rather than being shocked, he's fascinated. To his amazement, there is no blood. But you used only twenty needles. "What about the other ten needles?" he asks, suddenly realizing what the answer is. He begins to laugh, a deep chuckle. "Oh shit!" he moans. Then laughs again.

He guessed right: the last ten are for his cock. Pulling his soft cock up towards his belly you lay it against the board. Using the remaining needles, you pin the thin skin along his shaft to the board. As you work, you choose your inserting points very carefully, avoiding any obvious veins or visible blood vessels. This helps minimize any bleeding. He holds rock still for these needles, his fear and anticipation is held in check by the profound vision of his cock being pinned down!

The whole scene so far has taken almost a half an hour. Time – for both of you – has seemed both to fly and to stand still. Once you have finished your work, you remove your gloves and lift up a hand mirror for your friend to get a really good look. The scene overwhelms him.

"Get a picture!" he whispers. "I've gotta have a picture of this."

After taking a few Polaroids, you let him savor the feeling of the butterfly for a few moments, and then finally begin the process of removing the needles. For this you put on a fresh pair of gloves, and prepare several fresh alcohol swabs. You pull each needle out carefully and discard it into your hard plastic "sharps container," then swab the insertion site with the alcohol swab (such a nice little sting that makes!). After the final needle is removed, you again rest your forearm on his chest. The physical contact helps him come down from the amazing high he has been riding.

His cock and balls, other than being stained from the Betadine, look the same. Only a couple of the insertion points have bled, and you wipe away the tiny spots of blood with another alcohol swab. Tonight, he may have a few sore places and tiny bruises on his balls, but within a day or two there will be no evidence of the scene except in his memory. You tell him to wash his balls tonight, and again in the morning, and if he sees any red spots around the insertion points to clean them with alcohol and to apply some antibiotic cream to minimize the chances of infection.

In this scene, you were both torturer and doctor, tormentor and advisor. Edge play scenes like this provide a wonderful, thrilling sensation experience and an intense awareness of the paradox of BDSM, where tenderness and invasiveness, pain and pleasure, come together in a consensual, conscious, joyful exploration.

Babes In Toyland

Equipment
An appropriately noisy and motion-capable children's toy
Rope

Techniques
This scene is much like the rope cock and ball bondage described in "Double Your Pleasure," page 79. The variant here is in using a child's toy as the weight, rather than a conventional weight. See previous guidelines about choosing, winding, and removing rope in genital bondage.

In Context
Around Christmastime, many grown-up "boys" dream of all the great toys Santa will leave for them under the Christmas tree. That goes for their leather Daddies, too.

It's Christmas morning and your boy has gently nudged you awake, the aroma of fresh brewed coffee wafting over from the cup he's put on your bedside table. After getting up and putting on your robe, you shuffle off to the living room, where your boy has started a fire in the fireplace and set out a fine Christmas breakfast on the coffee table. After having breakfast, you both exchange a few gifts – soon you're on the floor in a pile of wrapping paper like a couple of kids.

One of the gifts he has given you is a brand new pair of leather cuffs. How thoughtful! A gift for you that you can use on him. You'd hate to just say thank you and then find out later that they didn't fit, so you tell him you want him to try them on for you. He's only too glad to oblige! Then, using the pair of eyelets you secured to the doorframe for just such an opportunity, you shackle his hands high above his head. He has a knowing smile as you urge his feet to the sides of the door jamb and order him to stay still.

Now you bring out a gift you have been saving – a bag from a local toy store. You taunt him with the gift, daring him to guess what it is. He can't stop giggling at the brightly colored sack. What could you have found for him at a kid's store?

From inside the sack you produce a gift-wrapped box. Again you give him a chance to guess, and tell him if he can't guess what it is; he will have to play with it by himself. He tries to look disappointed, but he can't help laughing. Through his chuckles he tells you he can't begin to guess, so you hold up the box to his face and tell him to pull the ribbon off with his teeth. While he does as you tell him, you take firm hold of his cock and balls and squeeze them. His laughter turns to a moan of pleasure as he fights with the ribbon. Once he has it off, you rip of the paper and reveal the surprise.

It's really a children's toy! A brightly-colored plastic sphere covered with rubber knobs, it looks a little like a land mine, but its purpose is not immediately evident. Putting it down, you pick up a length of rope that you had sealed inside the gift box. Wrapping it around the base of his cock, and then around the top of his scrotum, you proceed to tie a noose around his balls, the coils of rope pushing his balls down and stretching the skin of his sack until it shines like leather. You then tie off the rope around the base of his scrotum with a single knot. Making a loop with the ends of the rope, you pull it through a small metal eyelet you have previously attached to the spiky plastic ball. Knotting the rope, you let the ball hang between your boy's legs, setting him off into peals of laughter as he imagines how goofy he looks with his balls anchored to a bright plastic toy.

Holding your finger to your mouth, you shush him. "Listen," you say, because this little gift does more than just dangle and look silly. With the flick of a tiny switch, the ball starts gyrating and wiggling up and down, back and forth, bouncing and taking advantage of every bit of elasticity in the skin of your boy's balls. His laughter returns, but this time it sounds less cheerful and more maniacal. He loves ball weights, and the irregular tugging of the lightweight toy is really doing the trick.

For now, you make good on your promise to make him play with his new gift alone, and you sit back and relax, watching the ball as it bounces and your boy as he writhes. By the look of his rigid cock, he is doing just fine, and will continue to do so for the next fifteen minutes, until you decide you need to take a hand in the fun. It only takes a few dozen strokes to make him come, and between the groans and the giggles, you both know you'll remember this simple little Christmas toy for a long time to come.

Afterword

In sex as in medicine, the specialist gets fewer patients than the general practitioner. Cock and ball play is not the whole of my sexuality, or anybody's, and while I approach it with great enthusiasm, I also try to put it into perspective. There are so many other things to enjoy, and so many other things that can be incorporated into cock and ball play, to say nothing of the many ways that cock and ball play can be incorporated into other sex play.

The point is not merely to specialize, but to experiment, not merely to do one thing fantastically well but to explore your horizons, gaining experience and knowledge as you go and having a fabulous time while you do it. Having a fabulous time involves knowing yourself and your partners, techniques and toys, but it also means knowing laws and lo-

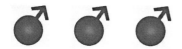

cal regulations to help ensure that your play does not land you or anyone else in trouble.

Where I live, in Texas, the law states that possessing two or more sex toys constitutes "intent to distribute," a crime punishable by fines and more hassle than any one person ever wants to have to handle. This raises some difficult questions, because what you may not think of as a sex toy someone else might, particularly if they wanted to give you a hard time legally. Is a napkin ring still a napkin ring if you use it as a cock ring, or does it become a sex toy? If zucchinis can be used as dildoes, do we have to stage a raid on the supermarket produce department?

Yes, I know it sounds silly, and it is. I have yet to figure out how sex toys constitute a major threat to the populace anyhow, but you never know when you're going to hear about a rapid rise in drive-by dildo-ings and forcible fitting of cock rings upon the unsuspecting. In Attleboro, Massachusetts, there are several consensual BDSM players who are as of this writing still fighting legal charges over, among other things, the use of a wooden kitchen spoon seized in a raid on a privately-held play party. There are many other highly publicized cases, including ones in other countries, such as the Spanner case in Britain.

I know it doesn't seem likely that anything like this would ever happen to you, but you never know, and I assure you that there are law enforcement authorities who will be more than willing to arrest on suspicion and let the courts sort it out. When our consensual sexual activities come under legal scrutiny, it is still very common to have lawyers, judges, and legislators characterize alternative sex play generally, and BDSM particularly, as obscenity, abuse, or assault.

I, and many other people, I am outraged that public officials still have the right to step into our bedrooms, our playrooms, our parties, and our lives. While I agree that abuse and assault are serious crimes and should indeed be prosecuted, safe, sane, and consensual sexuality, including BDSM, should not. But the onus for making sure that your sexuality does not become the focus of a legal case rests with you, not with the law. It is up to you to know the laws under which you live, and to help educate yourself and the people with whom you play as well as the general public about the differences between abuse and assault on the one hand and consensual BDSM activity on the other. We cannot count on other organizations to do this for us, we must do it for ourselves.

Our self-esteem, care, common sense, and intelligent compassion as leatherpeople will give us the strength, solidarity, and endurance to make this world a safe place for sexual exploration. It is my hope that everyone who reads this book will join me in taking steps to make their own sex life and sex play an expression of community, safety, and joy so that we will have a future in which the "differently pleasured" are not forced back into the closet, but accepted within the continuum of human diversity.

Other Books from Greenery Press

BDSM/KINK

The Bullwhip Book
Andrew Conway $11.95

The Compleat Spanker
Lady Green $12.95

Erotic Tickling
Michael Moran $13.95

Flogging
Joseph W. Bean $11.95

Intimate Invasions: The Ins and Outs of Erotic Enema Play
M.R. Strict $13.95

Jay Wiseman's Erotic Bondage Handbook
Jay Wiseman $16.95

The Loving Dominant
John Warren $16.95

Miss Abernathy's Concise Slave Training Manual
Christina Abernathy $12.95

The Mistress Manual: The Good Girl's Guide to Female Dominance
Mistress Lorelei $16.95

The Seductive Art of Japanese Bondage
Midori, photographed by Craig Morey $27.95

The Sexually Dominant Woman: A Workbook for Nervous Beginners
Lady Green $11.95

SM 101: A Realistic Introduction
Jay Wiseman $24.95

Training With Miss Abernathy: A Workbook for Erotic Slaves and Their Owners
Christina Abernathy $13.95

GENERAL SEXUALITY

Big Big Love: A Sourcebook on Sex for People of Size and Those Who Love Them
Hanne Blank $15.95

The Bride Wore Black Leather... And He Looked Fabulous!: An Etiquette Guide for the Rest of Us
Andrew Campbell $11.95

The Ethical Slut: A Guide to Infinite Sexual Possibilities
Dossie Easton & Catherine A. Liszt $16.95

A Hand in the Bush: The Fine Art of Vaginal Fisting
Deborah Addington
$13.95

Health Care Without Shame: A Handbook for the Sexually Diverse and Their Caregivers
Charles Moser, Ph.D., M.D. $11.95

The Lazy Crossdresser
Charles Anders $13.95

Look Into My Eyes: How to Use Hypnosis to Bring Out the Best in Your Sex Life
Peter Masters $16.95

Phone Sex
Miranda Austin $15.95

Photography for Perverts
Charles Gatewood $27.95

Sex Disasters... And How to Survive Them
C. Moser, Ph.D., M.D. and J. Hardy $16.95

Tricks... To Please a Man
Tricks... To Please a Woman
both by Jay Wiseman $14.95 ea.

Turning Pro: A Guide to Sex Work for the Ambitious and the Intrigued
Magdalene Meretrix $16.95

When Someone You Love Is Kinky
Dossie Easton & Catherine A. Liszt $15.95

FICTION

The 43rd Mistress: A Sensual Odyssey
Grant Antrews $11.95

... But I Know What You Want: 25 Sex Tales for the Different
James Williams $13.95

Haughty Spirit
Sharon Green $11.95

Love, Sal: letters from a boy in The City
Sal Iacopelli, ill. Phil Foglio $13.95

Murder At Roissy
John Warren $15.95

The Warrior Within
The Warrior Enchained   both by Sharon Green
$11.95 ea.

Please include $3 for first book and $1 for each additional book with your order to cover shipping and handling costs, plus $10 for overseas orders. VISA/MC accepted. Order from:

greenery press
3403 Piedmont Ave. #301, Oakland, CA 94611
toll-free 888/944-4434   http://www.greenerypress.com